Dash Diet Recipes

THE BEST DASH DIET COOKBOOK TO LOWER YOUR BLOOD PRESSURE, IMPROVE YOUR HEALTH, AND LOSE WEIGHT WITH QUICK AND EASY RECIPES

Charlotte E. Grey

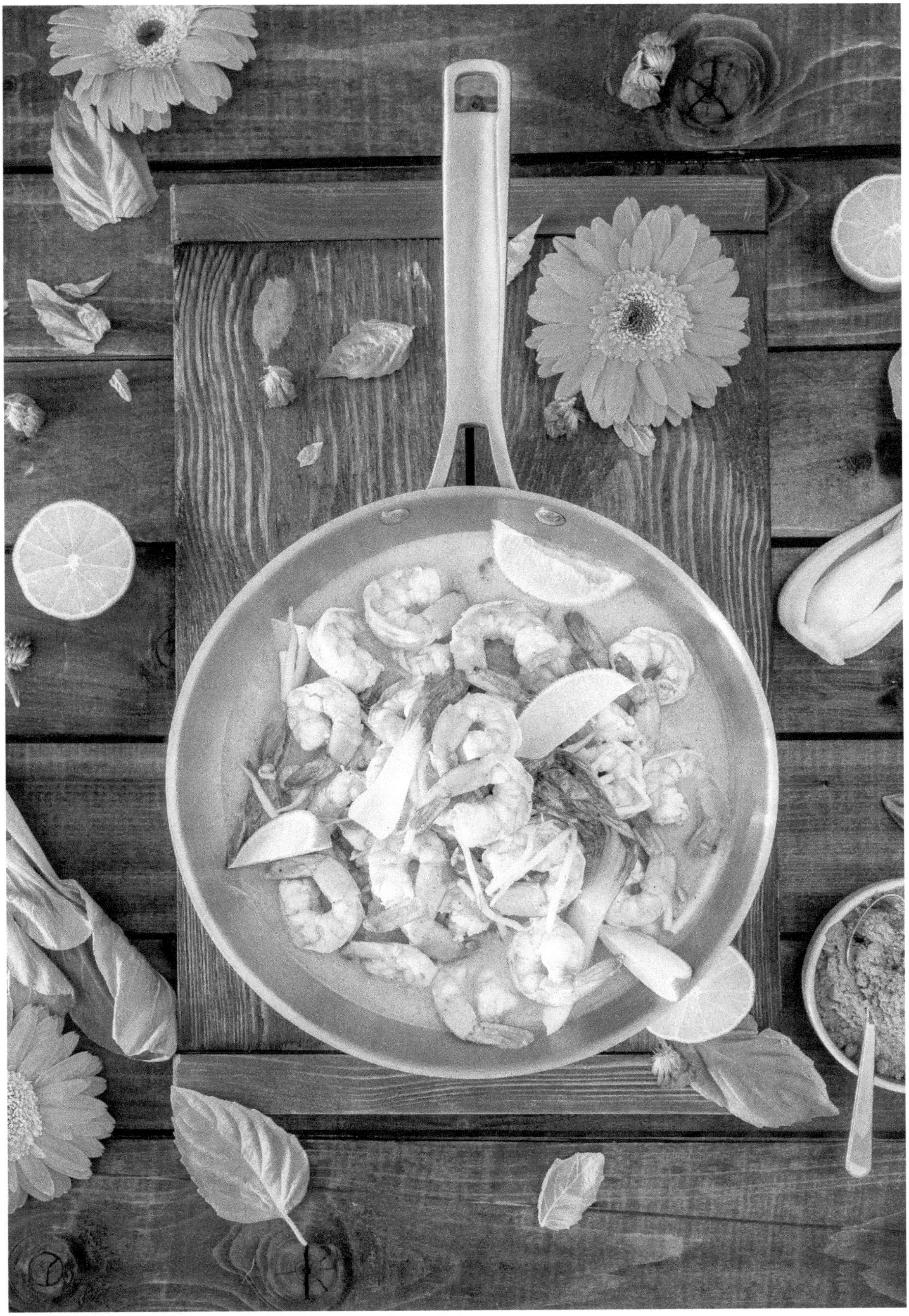

Table of Contents

Chapter 1: What is Dash Diet?

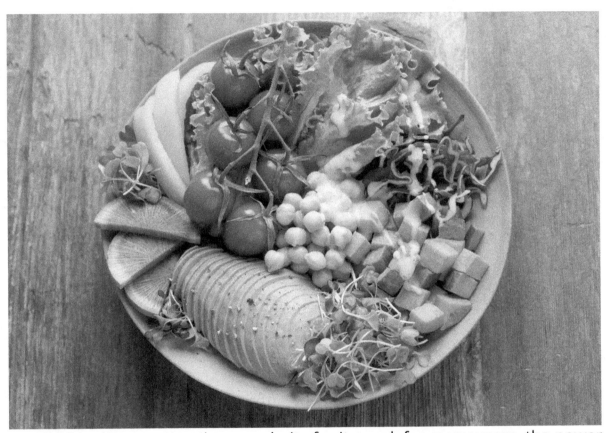

The DASH Diet is now attracting popularity for its work for many years, the power to lower blood pressure and the body's vulnerability to wide-ranging kinds of ailments. DASH stands for dietary approaches to stop hypertension, an originally developed routine offered to patients seeking to eliminate sodium in their foods; under the DASH Diet, the idea is that a lowered sodium intake contributes to lowered blood pressure, and this is also the ideal routine for those who strive to be safe and stop blood pressure. Except those who were brought on the DASH Diet in the process realized they had lost weight too! Therefore, the

DASH Diet was introduced to the community. In the 1990s, when the DASH diet was established, it initially incorporated a staple of carbohydrates and starchy foods.

Ultimately, it was changed to the shape that today we see a diet relying on an excess of fresh fruit and vegetables, low-fat meats, and nutritious proteins include seeds, beans, and nuts.

In addition, healthy whole grains like whole-wheat bread are permitted as part of the diet, but in moderation—the empty carbohydrates are used in standardized products. E.g., white bread and other items are cut out of the diet, seeing how they put on the calories and add to blood pressure. It has been shown by those who adhere closely to the DASH Diet to be one of the most effective ways to reduce lbs. And their bodies get all over better. Breakfast, lunch, and dinner are easy to prepare for: Food is incorporated with low-fat milk products, such as milk and yogurt, plenty of fresh fruit, leafy greens, such as spinach and vegetables such as broccoli, lean meats such as chicken and fish, and protein beans served, helping in weight loss.

The DASH Diet is typically split into two stages:

- Stage One. It lasts two weeks and is supposed to target abdominal fat.

- Stage Two. Takes in more Food, which was not permitted in the first two weeks and which is the longer-lasting. The stage is said to be the one on which dieters continue for the remainder of their lives. No wonder what the reason for starting the DASH Diet, the advantages of it is not possible to question this regiment, since they lead to a healthy body overall.

The DASH diet Eating Plan

The aim of the DASH diet eating plan is to include fresh fruits and vegetables, Low-fat dairy ingredients into the everyday diet, and lean forms of protein. It is directed at the amount of sodium and sodium, refined sugar, fat and red meat should be limited. Nutrition is full of nutrients, particularly potassium, which encourages low blood pressure. Magnesium, protein, fiber, and calcium.

The guidelines for regular servings focused on 2,000 calories per day are below. The National Institutes of Health established these guidelines.

Whole grains: 6-8 regular servings

Bread, cereals, pasta, quinoa, oats, rice, rye as well as wheat are included in this list.
It is advised that you should choose whole grains over white and processed grain.

Sample Serving:
- One bread slice
- One cereal ounce
- 1⁄2 cup of pasta or rice cooked
- Vegetables: 4–6 daily servings

This group contains asparagus, broccoli, sprouts from Brussels, carrots, celery, Green beans, vegetables with green leaves, Squash, spinach, sweet potatoes, kale, pumpkin, tomatoes, lettuce, peppers, potatoes, turnips, etc. as well as the veggies.

Sample Serving:
- 1 cup of leafy vegetation
- 1⁄2 cup of vegetables cooked or raw

- 1⁄2 cup of juice for vegetables
- Fruits: 4–6 regular servings

Included in this list are bananas, apples, cherries, dates, peaches, pears, raisins, grapes, grapefruit, lemons, mangoes, melons, strawberries, and melons Both watermelon and other fruits.

Sample Serving:
- One apple, peach, or pear medium
- 1⁄2 cup of fresh fruit, frozen or canned
- 1⁄4 fruit dried
- Dairy products: 2–3 regular servings

This group contains low-fat / non-fat milk, buttermilk, cheeses that are low-fat / non-fat, Low-fat / non-fat yogurt as well.

Sample Servings:
- 1 cup milk or yogurt (8 ounces)
- One and a half ounces of cheese
- Lean protein: between 3 and 6 servings a day

There are meats, poultry, fish, and eggs in this group. Pick lean meat cuts and strip the extra fat down. Remove the poultry skin.

Sample Serving:
- One egg
- One ounce of cooked meat (four ounces is around the size of a deck of cards to visualize.)

- Nuts, seeds, legumes: three to five servings a week

This group covers black beans, almonds, hazelnuts, kidney beans, legumes, pumpkin seeds, and sunflower seeds, split peas like other lentils, almonds Seeds, and legumes.

Sample Serving:

- 1/3 cup nuts (1 1/2 ounces)
- Two spoons of peanut butter
- Two spoons of sunflower seeds
- 1/2 cup of legumes cooked
- Oils and fats: 2-3 servings a day

Included in this group are coconut oil, ghee, margarine, olive oil, low-fat mayonnaise, oil, dressings for salads, and vegetable oils.

Sample Serving:

- One teaspoon of olive oil (better if extra virgin)
- One teaspoon of margarine
- One spoonful of mayonnaise
- Two tbsp of salad dressing
- Sweets and sugars: 5 or less week

This includes fruit flavored gelatins, candies, jelly, sorbets, maple syrup, and white or brown sugar.

Sample Serving:

- One spoonful of sugar

- One spoonful of jam
- 1⁄2 cup of sorbet

The chart below details the number of regularly prescribed servings for different servings. The amount of calories per day necessary depends on the number of calories consumed. Factors like your current age, weight, gender, and level of exercise.

FOOD GROUPS	SERVINGS/DAYS		
	1,600 calories/day	2,600 calories/day	3,600 calories/day
Grains	6	10–11	12–13
Vegetables	3–4	5–6	6
Fruits	4	5–6	6
Nonfat or low fat dairy products	2–3	3	3–4
Lean meats, poultry and fish	3–6	6	6–9
Nuts, seeds and legumes	3 week	1	1
Fats and oils	2	3	4
Sweets and sugars	0	less than 2	less than 2

Utensils & Cookware for DASH Diet

It will be easier to follow the DASH diet with your cookware and kitchen equipment. Items that are helpful include:

- Non-Stick Cookware: When sauteing meat or vegetables, non-stick kitchenware reduces the need to use oil or butter.

- Steamer for vegetables: A vegetable steamer that fits into the lower part of a pan makes it much easier to prepare vegetables without additional fat and calories, with a low nutrient deficit.

- A spice mill or press for garlic: These products make it easier for your food to add flavor and decrease your reliance on the saltshaker.

DASH diet, hypertension, and apnea for sleep

Hypertension is related to heart disease, diabetes, and several other concerns. Sleep apnea is less common but no less severe. The predominant symptom of sleep apnea is known to be snoring. Why is hypertension related to the DASH diet? It's really easy. Snore is an indication that oxygen is not appropriate. It keeps our arteries stronger so that they can carry blood, which increases blood pressure in part and may contribute to chronic hypertension further.

Cholesterol and glycemic levels decrease on the DASH diet, blood pressure is more regulated, snoring becomes quieter, and our overall health significantly changes. And without having any of the symptoms alluded to, you should try the diet. Supported by knowledgeable circles, it is considered one of the world's most healthy eating habits.

Chapter 2: Reduction in Salt Consumption

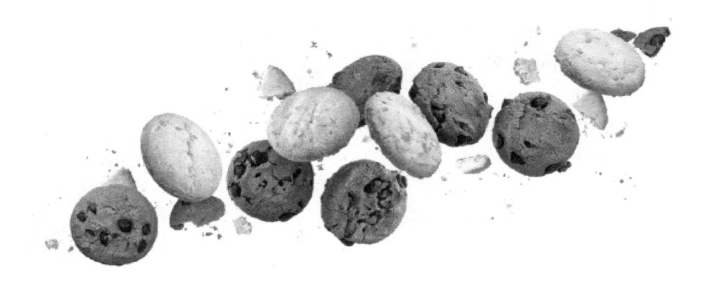

One of the main goals of the DASH diet is to drastically reduce the consumption of salt. Of course, man cannot live without salt. The human body contains around 150 to 300 grams of table salt. The amount of salt lost through sweating and other excretions must therefore be replaced. Salt supports the bone structure and digestion and it maintains the osmotic pressure in the vessels in order to maintain the water and nutrient levels. But nowadays our foods are filled with too salt - especially all finished products.

The extent to which increased salt consumption has a negative impact on health is currently the subject of intense discussion among experts, especially since excess salt is excreted by the body.

But studies from 1970 in Finland already show that too much salt causes blood pressure to skyrocket. It could be shown that the reduced consumption of salt by 30% could even reduce mortality from heart attacks by 80%.

A study on mice published in 2007 at the University Hospital in Heidelberg showed that a lot of salt increases blood pressure: "Salt promotes the formation of certain messenger substances in the muscles of blood vessels that cause the muscle cells to contract. The increased resistance in the blood vessels increases blood pressure. "The Heidelberg scientists therefore see considerable advantages in reducing the amount of salt in food compared to conventional drugs.

There is disagreement among scientists about how high the maximum amount of salt can be. While US experts recommend a maximum of 1.5 grams of salt per day, the recommendation of the German Nutrition Society is 6 grams per day and the upper limit is 10 grams per day. 6 grams are roughly equivalent to 1.20 teaspoons. However, this only applies to a healthy person who moves sufficiently and is physically active and excretes the salt again through sweating. For example, an athlete can tolerate more salt than someone who only moves moderately.

I recommend that you only look at these values as a rough guide and begin to control your salt consumption and gradually reduce it. Also keep in mind that the maximum amount of salt that you should consume depends on your individual body constitution and lifestyle.

Recommendation:

- Less is more! Therefore, pay more attention to your salt consumption in the future and reduce it step by step. The keyword is low-salt, but not salt-free!
- Avoid finished products (packaged food, pizza, French fries, chips, canned food, various meat and fish products, but also baked goods, etc.). If necessary, read the list of ingredients.
- If possible, use a natural salt substitute (herbs, etc.) in your meals
- Use low-water cooking methods such as stewing or steaming. This means that the food remains tastier and you don't need to salt it as much (see also tips on reducing salt consumption).

More vitamin E and minerals

The DASH diet is based on a variety of fruits and vegetables as well as whole grain products to provide the body with plenty of vitamins and minerals. Particular attention is paid to minerals such as magnesium and potassium, which help lower or improve blood pressure.

More healthy fats and oils

Fats are energy carriers and ensure that fat-soluble vitamins such as vitamins E, D and K can be absorbed by the body at all. Certain fatty acids, such as omega-3 and omega-6 fatty acids, are also essential, which means that we can only get them from food. Therefore, they should be on the regular meal plan. The omega-6/3 ratio plays an important role in health. Omega-3 fatty acids help to wisely maintain normal blood pressure levels. However, our diet often contains too little omega-3 fatty acids. Good sources of this are fatty fish such as herring, mackerel, salmon, and sardines.

This also applies to the use of oils. Z and healthy oils include virgin cold-pressed olive oil and coconut oil (in organic quality). Unlike olive oil, coconut oil can also be heated and used for frying and baking. The much-used sunflower oil, on the other hand, is less healthy because it only contains omega-6 fatty acids. This creates an imbalance in the omega-3 to omega-6 ratio. A ratio between 1: 2 and 1: 5 should be aimed for.

Ultimately, as with most other diets, the DASH diet should avoid unhealthy fats, especially trans fats, a subgroup of unsaturated fatty acids, and replace them with healthy fats such as those found in nuts, seeds and fish. Trans fatty acids come from industrial production and are, for example, contained in chips, baked goods, French fries, confectionery, pizza, etc.

More fiber
Fiber is an integral part of the DASH diet. A fiber-rich diet, whether through fruits, vegetables, grains and cereals, has a positive effect on blood pressure and the cardiovascular system.

In contrast to the low carb diet, grain can therefore be consumed. However, it is important to consume only wholesome grains (whole grain bread).

Egg whites / proteins
Proteins are an important part of the DASH diet and should be consumed in the form of beans, lentils, fish and soy products.

White instead of dark meat

Animal fat should be avoided as far as possible. It is high in cholesterol and saturated fat. Therefore, red meat should be avoided entirely if possible. Instead, white meat (chicken, turkey) can be put on the plate.

Avoid butter

Even if opinions differ widely about the consumption of butter, especially about its effect on the cholesterol level, the DASH diet specifies that butter should be avoided as far as possible and therefore butter no longer belongs in the refrigerator. Vegetable oils should serve as a substitute.

Now margarine is anything but healthy and therefore not an alternative in my opinion. I therefore recommend switching to ghee, the Ayurvedic butter. Ghee is pure butter fat and contains 70% saturated fatty acids. In Ayurveda, Ghee has been used for healing purposes for thousands of years. Studies have shown that ghee can even lower cholesterol and prevent diseases such as cardiovascular diseases. The advantage of ghee is that, unlike butter, it can be heated to a high temperature.

Low fat dairy products

The reduced-fat variant should always be preferred for dairy products (max. 1.5% fat content).

Less alcohol, caffeine and nicotine

Alcohol increases blood pressure. The DASH diet recommends avoiding alcohol, beverages containing caffeine and nicotine as much as possible in order to reduce blood pressure.

If you don't want to go without your coffee, you should enjoy it with as little or no sugar as possible.

It is also known that smoking increases the risk of heart attacks and strokes. So - if you haven't already done so - put an end to the glowing stick!

Reduction of industrial sugar (granulated sugar)

Most people should know by now that too much sugar is not healthy. The DASH diet does not completely exclude sugar, after all, fresh and dried fruits are an important part of this diet and of course they also contain sugar (fructose).

What has a negative effect on blood pressure, however, is pure industrial sugar. This can quickly increase blood pressure and should therefore be avoided as far as possible. The best way to regulate daily sugar consumption is to avoid sweets and finished products.

A possible alternative to industrial sugar, which is not exactly cheap, is coconut blossom sugar, which, despite its calories, keeps the blood sugar level more constant.

Check daily calorie intake

The DASH diet recommends a calorie intake between 1,500 and 2,300 kcal per day. If you want to lose weight, you should limit the value to 1,500 kcal per day. Of course, this is only a guideline and depends on the basal metabolic rate, age, body weight and size, muscular mass, gender and health status. You can find a variety of calculators on the Internet to determine your calorie requirement (e.g. with Fit-for-Fun, Smart Calculator).

Summary

- Use low-salt and low-fat foods
- Avoid finished products
- Avoid industrial sugar (choose natural sugar substitutes)
- Lots of fresh vegetables and fruits
- Healthy fats and oils (no trans fats)
- Little alcohol and caffeine
- No nicotine
- High fiber foods
- Choose whole grain products
- Nuts, seeds and beans as part of meals
- Low fat dairy products
- Reduce animal fat (opt for white meat)
- Replace butter with ghee (clarified
- Fish
- Plenty of water
- Pay attention to maximum calorie intake

Chapter 3: Breakfast Recipes

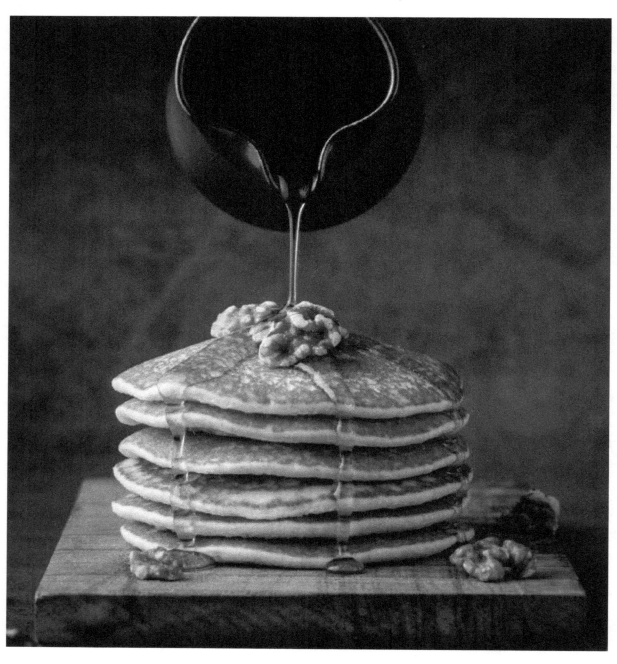

Almond Butter and Banana Toasts

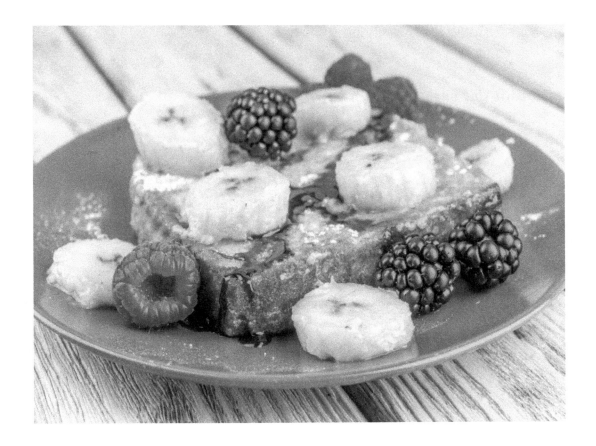

PREP TIME: 7 MINS

COOK TIME: 5MINS

SERVINGS: 1

Ingredients

- 2 slices of 100% whole wheat bread
- Almond butter 2 tbsp

- One tiny banana, cut

- 1/8 tbps of cinnamon ground

How To:

1. Toast the bread and spread the almond butter evenly on each piece. Place the banana slices on top, and sprinkle them with cinnamon.

Nutrition (amount per serving):

484 Calories, Fat 21 g, sodium 402 mg, potassium 56 g

British Muffin

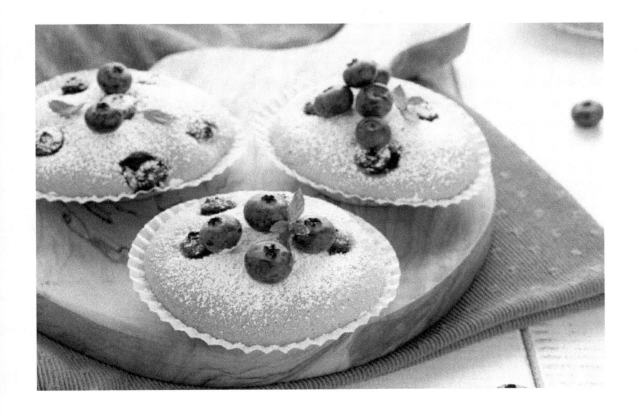

PREP TIME: 5 MINS

COOK TIME: 5 MINS

SERVINGS: 1

Ingredients

- 100 percent whole wheat English muffin
- One cup of cream cheese (reduced fat)
- Four strawberries, cut thinly
- 1/2 cup of crushed blueberries

How To:

1. Cut the English muffins into halves and toast them. Spread the cream cheese on each toasted half, equally, and cover with the fruit.

Nutrition:

Calories 231, Total Fat 4 g, Sodium 270 m, Protein 8 g, Calcium 5%

Black Bean Brownies

PREP TIME: 5 MINS

COOK TIME: 20 MINS

SERVINGS: 2

Ingredients

- 1 1/2 cups of black beans, washed, rinsed (1 15-ounce can)
- 2 tablespoons of cocoa powder
- 1/2 cup of quick oats
- 1/4 teaspoon of salt
- 1/3 cup of pure maple syrup or agave, or honey
- 2 tablespoons of sugar
- 1/4 cup of coconut oil or vegetable oil
- 2 teaspoons of pure vanilla extract
- 1/2 teaspoon of baking powder
- 1/2-2/3 cup of chocolate chips

How To:

1. Preheat oven to 350 °F.

2. Blend together all ingredients, except the chocolate chips, until absolutely smooth. Blend well. (Food processor works best for texture. A blender is perfect if needed.)

3. Add chocolate chips and pour them into an eight-in-eight grated plate. Optional: Sprinkle on top the extra chocolate chips.

4. Cook for about 15–18 minutes. Let chill down for at least 10 minutes before cutting (yields around 9–12 squares). If they look a little undercooked, you can put them overnight in the fridge, and they'll be firmed up.

Nutrition (Per Serving)

Calories: 201, Fat: 5g, Carb: 38g, Protein: 4g, Sodium 7mg

Shameless Banana Split

PREP TIME: 5 MINS

COOK TIME: 0 MINS

SERVINGS: 2

Ingredients

- 1 banana, sliced in half lengthwise
- 1/2 cup of cottage cheese
- 1/2 cup of mixed berries
- 1 teaspoon of ground flaxseed
- 1 teaspoon of chia seed
- 1 tablespoon of chopped walnuts.

How To:

1. Put banana slices into a pot. Add cottage cheese scoops in the middle.

2. Top with berries and flaxseed and garnish with chia seeds and walnuts.

Nutrition (Per Serving)

- Calories: 138
- Fat: 3g
- Carb: 29g
- Protein: 1g
- Sodium 4mg

Daphne Oz's Sugar Break Banana Bread

PREP TIME: 5 MINS

COOK TIME: 45 MINS

SERVINGS: 4

Ingredients

- 4 medium bananas, mashed
- 1 egg
- 1 egg yolk
- 1 tsp of vanilla extract
- 1 stick of unsalted butter, melted
- 1 cup of all-purpose whole grain flower
- 1/2 cup of cocoa powder
- 1 tsp of baking soda
- 1/8 tsp salt
- 1/2 cup of semisweet chocolate chips
- 2 tbsp of black sesame seeds (optional)

How To:

1. Preheat oven to 350 °F.
2. Combine mashed bananas, egg & egg yolk, and vanilla in a medium-sized container. When the melted butter has cooled slightly, whisk into a banana mixture.
3. Whisk the flour, cocoa powder, brown sugar (if used), baking soda, and salt together in a separate container. Gently mix the dry ingredients into a mixture with the bananas until smooth.
4. Pour flour into a loaf pan (prepared with butter). Sprinkle with the sesame seeds on top (if used). Bake for 45-50 minutes, until the inserted toothpick (or knife), comes out clean.

5.   Allow it to cool for a few minutes before serving.

Nutrition (Per Serving)

*   Calories: 145, Fat: 4.5g, Carb: 19g, Protein: 8.5g, Sodium 77mg

Guilt-Not Chocolate Avocado Mousse

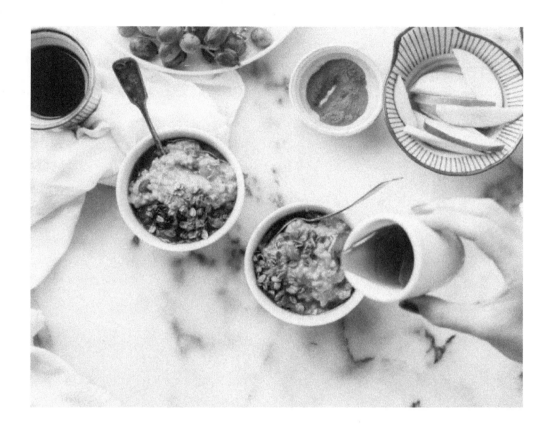

PREP TIME: 10 MINS

COOK TIME: 0 MINS

SERVINGS: 2

Ingredients

- 1 large avocado (very ripe)
- 1/4 cup of almond milk or coconut milk
- 2 tablespoon of coconut oil
- 1/4 cup of cocoa or cacao powder

- 1 teaspoon of vanilla extract.

How To:

1. Blend all ingredients until creamy.

2. Chill for few hours in the refrigerator or better, overnight.

Nutrition (Per Serving)

- Calories: 467

- Fat: 41g

- Carbohydrates: 3g

- Protein: 20g

Greek Yogurt Chocolate Chip Cookie Dough Dip

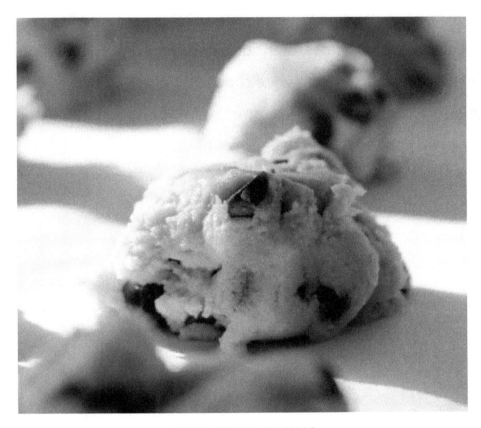

PREP TIME: 5 MINS

COOK TIME: 0 MINS

SERVINGS: 4

Ingredients

- 1 cup of simple Greek yogurt
- 1/4 cup creamy organic peanut, cashew or almond butter
- 1/2 tsp pure vanilla extract

- 1/4 tsp of kosher salt
- Stevia or honey, to taste
- 1/2 cup mini dark chocolate chips
- apple slices, to serve

How To:

1. Combine the Greek yogurt, almond butter, vanilla extract, and kosher salt in a medium bowl, then whisk until smooth.

2. Sweeten with Stevia to taste, then stir in chocolate chips. (There is less sugar in dark chocolate chips than milk or white chocolate)

3. Serve as a dip with apple slices, or enjoy with a spoon! (Remember, for a frozen yogurt treat, pop the dips in the freezer.)

Nutrition (Per Serving)

- Calories: 250
- Fat: 13g
- Carbohydrates: 40g

Peach and Granola Parfait

PREP TIME: 5 MINS

COOK TIME: 0 MINS

SERVINGS: 4

Ingredients

- Plain low-fat Greek yogurt - 1 cup Honey – 2 Tbsp.

- Vanilla extract – ¼ tsp.

- No-salt-added granola – 8 Tbsp. Ripe peaches – 4, diced

How To:

1. Stir the honey, yogurt, and vanilla in a bowl.

2. For each serving, in a large parfait glass, layer 1 tbsp. granola, 2 tbsp. yogurt, and 1/8 of the diced peaches, then repeat.

3. Serve.

Nutrition (Per Serving)

- Calories: 145

- Fat: 45.5g

- Carb: 19g

- Protein: 8.5g

- Sodium 247mg

Pear Crumble

PREP TIME: 5 MINS

COOK TIME: 30 MINS

SERVINGS: 2

Ingredients

- Cooking spray (better if low fat)
- 5 chopped ripe pears 2 tsp. of honey
- 1 tbsp. of fresh lemon juice 2 tsp. of cornstarch
- ½ tsp. of grated nutmeg
- 1 cup - granola with no added salt

How To:

1. Preheat the oven to 350F. Grease a baking dish with cooking spray.
2. Mix the honey, pears, lemon juice, cornstarch, and nutmeg in the baking dish.
3. Bake for 30 minutes, (stirring after 15 minutes). or until pears are tender. Remove.
4. Sprinkle the granola over the pear mixture.
6. Return to the oven and bake just to heat the granola, about 5 minutes.
7. Cool and serve.

Nutrition (Per Serving)

- Calories: 201
- Fat: 5g
- Carb: 38g
- Protein: 4g

- Sodium 7mg

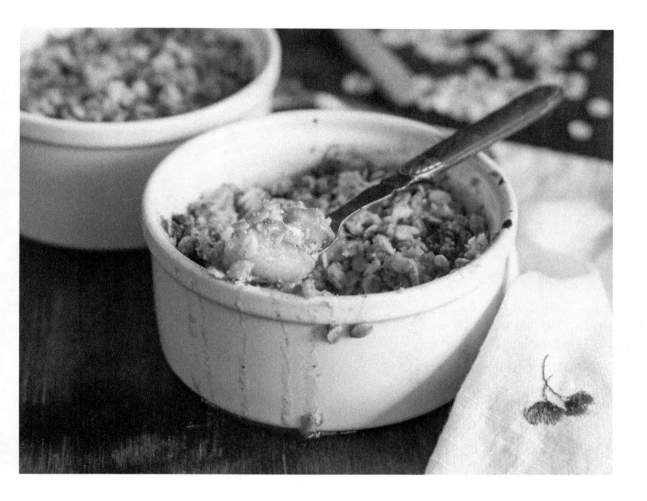

Roasted Pineapple covered in Maple Syrup

PREP TIME: 15 MINS

COOK TIME: 20 MINS

SERVINGS: 2

Ingredients

- Ripe pineapple – ½ cut into wedges
- Maple syrup – ¼ cup
- Unsalted butter (melted) – 1 tbsp.

How To:

1. Preheat the oven to 425F.

2. Working with 1 pineapple wedge at a time, use a paring knife to cut the flesh from the rind in one piece. Cut the flesh vertically into 5 large chunks, keeping them nestled in the rind.

3. Arrange the pineapple wedges in a baking dish and spray with oil.

4. Roast for 15 minutes.

5. Whisk together the maple syrup and butter in a bowl.

6. Brush the mixture over the pineapple and bake for 5 minutes more.

7. Transfer to serving plates. Drizzle with any remaining liquid from the baking dish.

Nutrition (Per Serving)

- Calories: 138, Fat: 3g, Carb: 29g, Protein: 1g, Sodium 4mg

Fresh Strawberries in Chocolate Dip

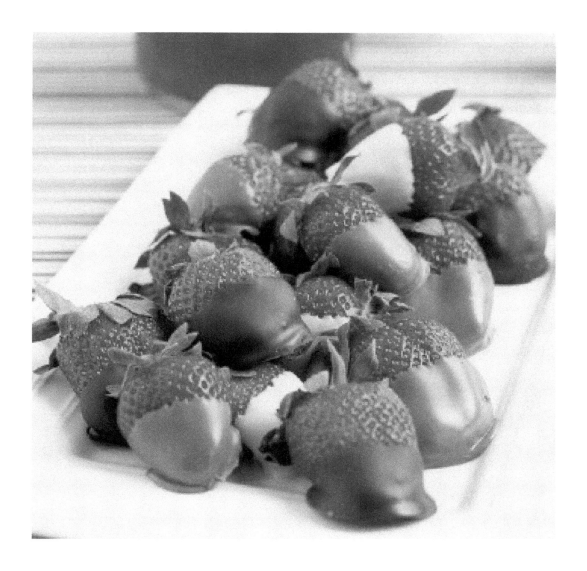

PREP TIME: 15 MINS

COOK TIME: 10 MINS

SERVINGS: 4

Ingredients

- Low-fat canned evaporated milk – ½ cup
- Bittersweet chocolate – 5 ounces, finely chopped
- Strawberries – 24, un-hulled

How To:

1. Bring the milk to a simmer in a saucepan.

2. Remove from heat and add chocolate. Let it stand until chocolate softens, about 3 minutes. Then start whisking until smooth.

3. Divide the chocolate mixture among four small bowls.

4. Serve the strawberries with the chocolate mixture for dipping.

Nutrition (Per Serving)

- Calories: 229

- Fat: 14g

- Carb: 28g

- Protein: 5g

- Sodium 36mg

Fresh Strawberries and Honey in a bed of yogurt

PREP TIME: 5 MINS

COOK TIME: 0 MINS

SERVINGS: 4

Ingredients

- 1 cup of quartered fresh strawberries
- 4 teaspoons of honey
- 3 cups plain lowfat yogurt 4 Tablespoons of toasted,
- and cut almonds

How To:

1. Clean and cut strawberries into quarters, and put on the side for later.

2. Scoop ¾ cup of yogurt into 4 small bowls. Divide the strawberries equally among the bowls. Top each bowl with 1 teaspoon of hone and then with 1 tablespoon toasted almonds pieces. Serve right away.

Tips:

New organic strawberries are normally sweet and require next to nothing else . Try to opt for this type of sweet crisp natural products and match them with low-fat or no-fat yogurt.

Nutrition (Per Serving)

- Calories: 250, Fat: 13g, Carbohydrates: 40g

Chapter 4: Side Dishes & Appetizers Recipes

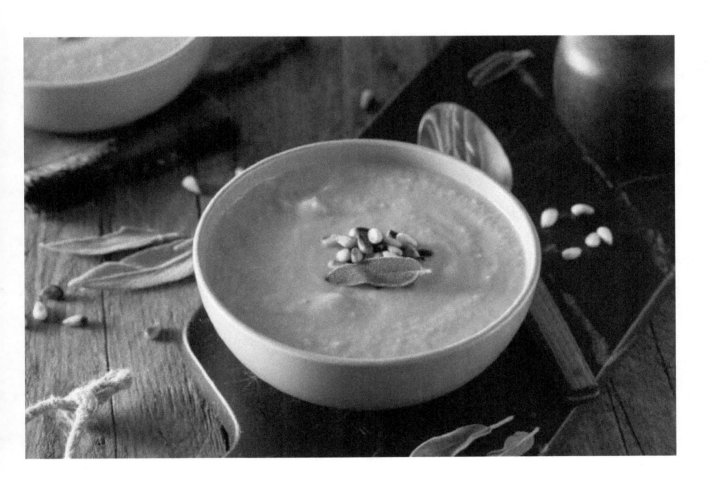

The Homey Carrots Blend

PREP TIME: 10 MINS

COOK TIME: 40 MINS

SERVINGS: 6

Ingredients

- 15 carrots, cut in half longitudinally
- Two teaspoons of sugar from coconut
- Olive oil ¼ cup
- ½ tsp dry rosemary,
- ½ tsp crushed garlic
- A squeeze of black pepper

How To:

1. Combine the carrots and the sugar, oil, rosemary, garlic powder, and black pepper in a cup, swirl properly, scatter on a rimmed baking sheet, put in the oven, and bake for 40 minutes at 400 °Fahrenheit

2. As a side dish, split across trays and eat.

3. Enjoy!

Nutrition:

Calories 211, fat 2g, fiber 6g, carbs

14g, Protein 8g

Asparagus on the Grill

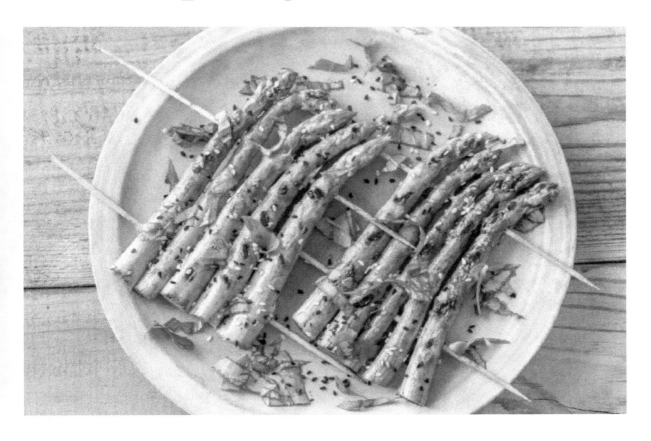

PREP TIME: 10 MINS

COOK TIME: 6 MINS

SERVINGS: 4

Ingredients

- Asparagus two pounds, cut
- Olive oil two tablespoons
- A pinch of black pepper and salt

How To:

1. Season the asparagus with salt, pepper and oil.

2. Put the asparagus over medium-high heat on the hot oven grill, cook around each

side for three minutes, or until they start blackening.

3.   Serve warm.

Nutrition:

Calories 172, fat 4g, protein 7g, carbs 14g, Protein 8g

Roasted Carrots

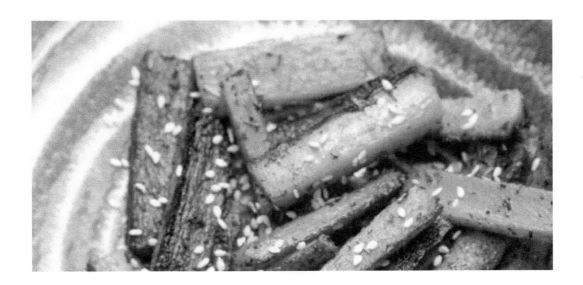

PREP TIME: 15 MINS

COOK TIME: 30 MINS

SERVINGS: 4

Ingredients

- Two pounds of diced carrots
- A squeeze of black pepper
- Olive oil 3 tablespoons
- Cut 2 teaspoons of parsley

How To:

1. On a rimmed baking sheet, arrange the carrots, season with black pepper and oil, turn, put in the oven, and cook for thirty min at 400 ° Fahrenheit.

2. Add in the parsley. Mix and serve as a side dish on plates.

3. Enjoy!

Nutrition:

Calories 177, fat 3g, fiber 6g, carbs 14g, Protein 6g

Oven Asparagus

PREP TIME: 10 MINS

COOK TIME: 25 MINS

SERVINGS: 4

Ingredients

- Two pounds of asparagus shaved
- Olive oil 3 tablespoons
- Black pepper to taste
- Two tsp of sweet paprika
- 1 teaspoon of seeds with sesame

How To:

1. Place the asparagus on a rimmed baking sheet, add oil, black pepper, and paprika.

2. Mix well, put the tray in the oven, and cook for 25 minutes at 400 ° Fahrenheit

3. Split the asparagus into bowls, scatter on top with the sesame seeds, and offer as a side dish.

4. Enjoy!

Nutrition:

Calories 190, fat 4g, fiber 8g, carbs

11g, Protein 5g

Potato Blend

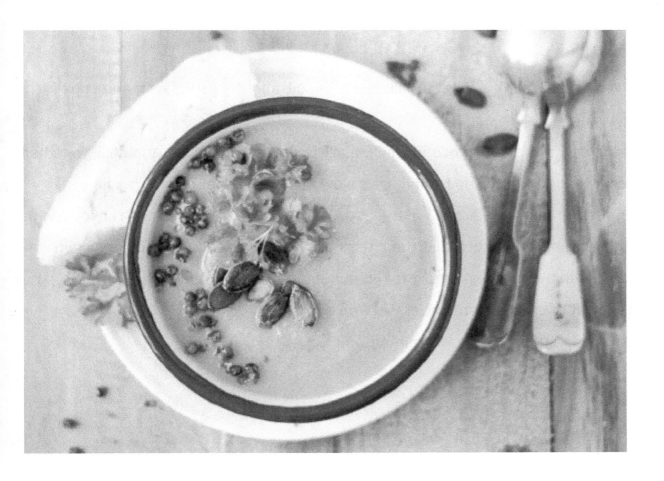

PREP TIME: 15 MINS

COOK TIME: 1 HOUR

SERVINGS: 8

Ingredients

- Six potatoes, cut and peeled
- 2 cloves of garlic, finely chopped
- Extra virgin olive oil 2 tablespoons
- One and 1⁄2 cups of coconut milk
- 1⁄4 cup of coconut milk
- Thyme 1 cup, diced
- 1⁄4 teaspoon of nutmeg

- A handful of dry chili flakes
- Low-fat cheddar 1 and 1/2 cups, crushed
- 1/2 cup low-fat, grated parmesan

How To:

1. Over a moderate fire, heat a skillet with the oil, add the garlic, swirl and cook for 1 minute.
1. Bring coconut cream, coconut milk, pieces of thyme, nutmeg, and chili, together and whisk. Bring to a boil, minimize to low flame, and cook for 10 minutes.
2. In a casserole tray, place 1/3 of the potatoes, insert 1/3 of the cream, replicate with the remaining potatoes and the cream, scatter the cheddar on top, seal with tin foil, put in the oven, and roast for 45 minutes at 375 °Fahrenheit
3. Take out of the oven and cover with the parmesan.
4. Bake it again for another 20 minutes.

Nutrition:

Calories 224, fat 8g, fiber 9g, carbs 16g, protein 15g

Simply Brussels Sprouts

PREP TIME: 5 MINS

COOK TIME: 20 MINS

SERVINGS: 6

Ingredients

- Two pounds of fresh sprouts Brussels, cut in half
- Olive oil 2 tablespoons
- A squeeze of black pepper
- Sesame Oil 1 tbsp
- Two cloves of garlic, diced
- 1/2 cup of coconut amino
- Two teaspoons of apple vinegar cider
- 1 tbsp of sugar coconut
- Two teaspoons of sauce with chili
- A pinch of flakes of red pepper
- Seeds of sesame for serving

How To:

1. Spread the sprouts on a paneled roasting pan, bring the black pepper, garlic, aminos, olive oil, the sesame oil, vinegar, coconut sugar, chili sauce, and pepper flakes, toss well, incorporate in the oven and bake at 425 °F for 20 minutes.

2. Distribute the sprouts among plates, sprinkle on top with sesame seeds, and use it as a side dish.

Nutrition:

Calories 176, fat 3g, fiber 6g, carbs 14g, protein 9g

Chapter 5: Chicken Recipes

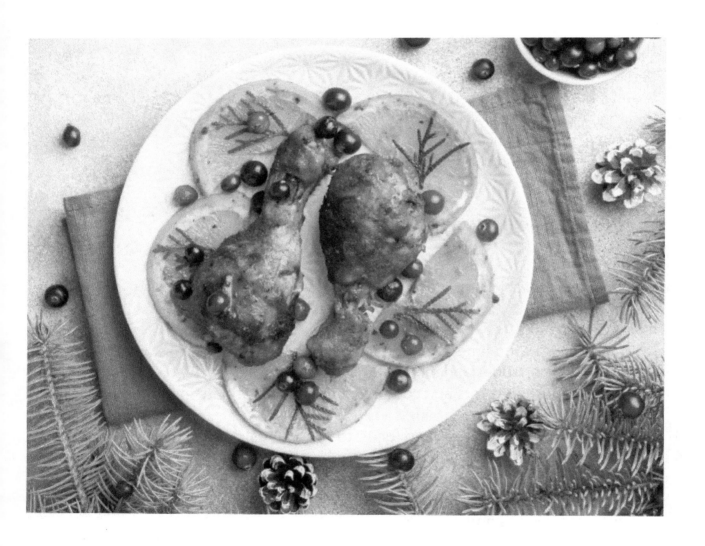

Tequila Chicken & Peppers

PREP TIME: 10 MINS

COOK TIME: 6 – 7 HOURS

SERVINGS: 4

Ingredients

- Lime juice – 1 cup
- Tequila – 1/3 cup
- Extra virgin olive oil
- Garlic – 3 cloves, chopped
- Green bell pepper – 1, diced
- Chopped fresh cilantro – ¼ cup
- Red bell pepper – 1, diced
- Agave nectar – 1 Tbsp.
- Onion – 1, diced
- Black pepper - ½ tsp.
- Non-fat sour cream – ½ cup
- Cumin – 1 tsp.
- Ground coriander – ½ tsp.
- Boneless, skinless chicken breasts – 4

How To:

1. In a bowl, add the lime juice, tequila garlic, cilantro, agave nectar, black pepper, cumin, and coriander and mix well.
2. Add the chicken breasts and coat well. Cover and marinate in the for least 6 hours (in the refrigerator).
3. Heat the grill. Cook the chicken for 10 to 15 minutes per side, or no longer pink.
4. Meanwhile, heat the oil in a pan.
5. Add the pepper and onion. Stir-fry for 5 minutes. Remove from heat. Remove chicken from grill.
6. Serve with veggies and sour cream.

Nutrition:

Calories: 259, Fat: 3g, Carb: 18g, Protein: 28g, Sodium 118mg

Chicken and Onion Mix

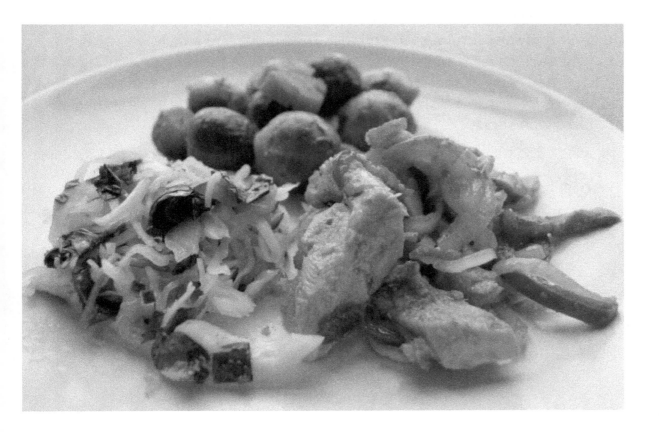

PREP TIME: 10 MINS

COOK TIME: 1 HOUR

SERVINGS: 4

Ingredients
- Olive oil 3 tablespoons
- One yellow onion, sliced roughly
- Thyme 2 tablespoons, diced
- Two cloves of garlic, diced
- A squeeze of black pepper
- Four skinless, boneless and cut into cubes chicken breasts
- Oregano 1/2 tsp, dry
- 1 and 1/2 cup of low-sodium stock of beef
- 1 tsp parsley, minced

How To:

1. Warm a pan over medium-low heat with two tablespoons of olive oil, introduce the onion, black pepper, and thyme, toss and simmer for 24 minutes.
2. Add garlic and cook for another 1 minute, then move it to a dish.
3. Empty the skillet, warm it over medium-high heat with the remaining oil, insert the chicken, black pepper, and oregano, stir and bake for another 8 minutes.
4. Incorporate beef, add parsley and onion blend, toss, boil for ten minutes, divide into bowls, and serve.

Nutrition:

Calories 231, fat 4g, fiber 7mg, carbs 14mg, protein 15g

Honey Crusted Chicken

PREP TIME: 10 MINS

COOK TIME: 25 MINS

SERVINGS: 2

Ingredients
- Saltine crackers – 8, (2-inch square each) crushed
- Paprika – 1 tsp.
- Chicken breasts – 2, boneless, skinless (4-ounce each)
- Honey – 4 tsp.
- Cooking spray to grease a baking sheet

How To:
1. Preheat the oven to 375F.
2. In a bowl, mix crushed crackers and paprika. Mix well.
3. In another bowl, add honey and chicken. Coat well.
4. Add to the cracker mixture and coat well.
5. Place the chicken in the prepared baking sheet.
6. Bake for 20 to 25 minutes.
7. Serve.

Nutrition:
Calories: 219, Fat: 3g, Carb: 21g, Protein: 27g, Sodium 187mg

Creamy Lemon Chicken Parmesan

PREP TIME: 10 MINS

COOK TIME: 25 MINS

SERVINGS: 4

Ingredients

- cup of all-purpose flour
- 2 large sized eggs, beaten
- ¾ cup of whole-wheat panko breadcrumbs
- ½ cup of grated Parmesan cheese, divided
- 1 teaspoon of Italian seasoning
- 1 teaspoon of garlic powder
- 4 4-ounce of chicken breast cutlets
- 3 tablespoons of extra-virgin olive oil, divided
- 2 cloves garlic, minced
- 1 cup of low-sodium chicken broth
- ¼ cup of lemon juice
- ¼ teaspoon of salt
- ½ cup of half-and-half
- ¼ cup of chopped fresh parsley

How To:

1. Preheat oven to 400 tiers F. Place flour in a shallow dish. Place overwhelmed eggs in every other shallow dish. Mix panko, 1/4 cup Parmesan, Italian seasoning and garlic powder in a 3rd shallow dish. Working with one at a time, coat every cutlet in flour, shaking off the excess. Transfer to the egg combination and turn to coat. Transfer to the panko aggregate and turn to coat. Reserve 1 tablespoon of the flour

(it'll be cooked later) in a small bowl. Discard any ultimate flour, egg and panko mixture.

2. Heat 1 tablespoon oil in a big skillet at medium-high temperature. Add 2 cutlets and cook, flipping once, until golden, 1 to 2 minutes according to side. Transfer to a huge baking sheet. Reduce warmth to medium and add any other 1 tablespoon oil to the pan. Add the closing cutlets and cook, flipping once, till golden on both sides, 1 to two minutes in step with side. Place   it to the baking sheet. Bake the cutlets until cooked throughout, about 10 minutes.

3. Meanwhile, wipe out the pan. Add the last 1 tablespoon oil and warmth over medium-high warmth pan. Add garlic and cooking, mixing, until fragrant, approximately 30 sec.

    Add broth, lemon juice and salt to the pan. Bring to a boil. Whisk half of-and-half of into the reserved 1 tablespoon flour. Add to the broth combi nation and cook, stirring frequently, until reduced by approximately half and thickened sufficient to coat the returned of a spoon, 8 to 10 minutes. Remove from heat.

4. Transfer the cutlets to a large platter. Sprinkle with the sauce and top with the ultimate 1/4 cup Parmesan and parsley.

Nutrition:
Calories: 219, Fat: 3g, Carb: 21g, Protein: 27g, Sodium 187mg

Smooth Chicken Cream

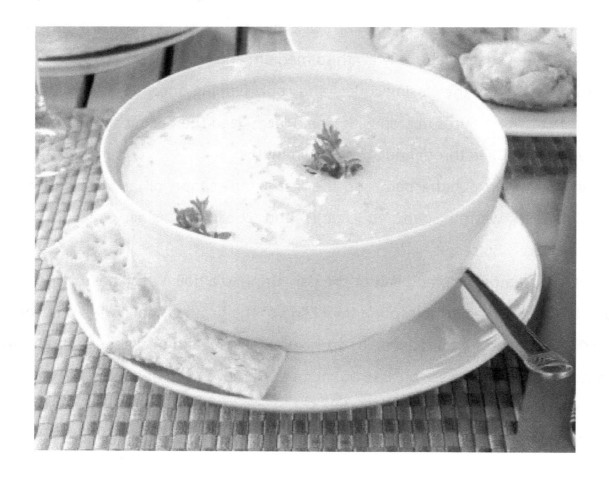

PREP TIME: 20 MINS

COOK TIME: 20 MINS

SERVINGS: 4

Ingredients

- Two breasts of chicken, boneless, skinless & sliced into pieces
- One chopped yellow onion
- Olive oil, 2 tablespoons
- One clove of garlic, diced
- Twelve ounces of zucchini, in cubes
- Two bits of carrots, minced
- To the taste, black pepper

- Fourteen ounces of coco-milk
- Seventeen ounces of chicken stock with reduced sodium

How To:
1. Over medium-high pressure, heat a pan with the oil, add the garlic and onion, mix and simmer for five minutes.
2. Include the carrots, chicken, zucchini, chicken stock & black pepper, whisk, bring to a boil, lower the heat to mild and boil for fifteen minutes.
3. Include the milk, move the soup to the mixer, pulse, ladle into the bowls of soup and eat.

Nutrition:
Calories 210, fat 7g, fiber 4mg, carbs 15mg, protein 12mg

Salsa Chicken

PREP TIME: 10 MINS

COOK TIME: 1 HOUR

SERVINGS: 4

Ingredients
- Sixteen ounces Salsa Verde canned
- To the taste, black pepper
- Olive oil,1 tablespoon
- One and 1⁄2 cups cheddar cheese fat-free, diced
- 1⁄4 cup minced parsley
- Juice of 1 lime
- Chicken breast 1 pound, skinless and boneless

How To:

1. Place the salsa in a baking dish, cover it with chicken, add oil, black pepper, lime juice, cover it with cheese, place it in the oven at 400.
2. Cook for 1 hour.
3. Spray on top of cilantro, split it all between plates and serve.

Nutrition:
- Calories 250
- fat 1g
- fiber 4mg
- carbs 14mg
- protein 12g

Chapter 6: Red Meat Recipes

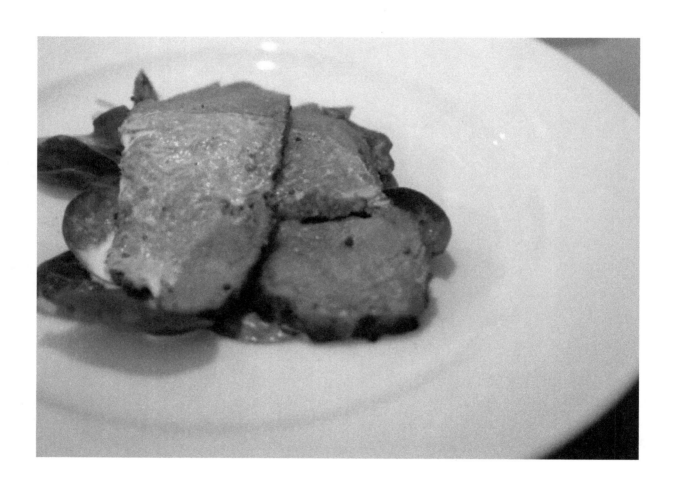

Roasted Pork in Herbs

PREP TIME: 25 MINS

COOK TIME: 1 HOUR

SERVINGS: 6

Ingredients
- Boneless pork loin roast – 2 lbs.
- Garlic – 3 cloves, minced
- Dried rosemary – 1 Tbsp.
- Dried thyme – 1 tsp.
- Dried basil – 1 tsp.
- Salt – ¼ tsp.
- Olive oil – ¼ cup
- White wine – ½ cup
- Pepper to taste

How To:
1. Preheat the oven to 350F.
2. Crush the garlic with thyme, rosemary, basil, salt, and pepper, making a paste. Set aside.
3. Use a knife to pierce meat several times.
4. Press the garlic paste into the slits.
5. Rub the meat with the rest of the garlic mixture and olive oil.
6. Place pork loin into the oven, turning and basting with pan liquids, until the pork reaches 145F, about 1 hour. Remove the pork from the oven.
7. Place the pan over heat and add white wine, stirring the brown bits on the bottom.
8. Top roast with sauce.
9. Serve.

Nutrition:
Calories: 464, Fat: 20.7g, Carb: 2.4g, Protein: 59.6g, Sodium 279mg

Pork and Frijoles Stew

PREP TIME: 10 MINS

COOK TIME: 1 HOUR 10 MINS

SERVINGS: 4

Ingredients

- Two pounds, cut and cubed pork butt
- Olive oil, 1 and 1⁄2 teaspoons
- Two sliced eggplants,
- One chopped yellow onion
- One bell pepper red, minced
- Three cloves of garlic, diced
- 1 tbsp of dried thyme
- Two teaspoons of dry sage,
- Four ounces of canned white beans, incorporated without salt, drained and rinsed.
- One cup low-sodium stock of chicken
- Twelve ounces of zucchini, chopped
- Two tablespoons of tomato paste

How To:
1. Put an oiled pan over medium-high heat. Once hot put the pork in it and let it brown for five minutes.
2. Add the onion, thyme, bell pepper, garlic, sage, and eggplants, swirl, and roast for another five minutes.
3. Include the beans, tomato paste, and stock, lower the heat and let it boil covered for 50 minutes.
4. Add the zucchinis, flip, fry for 10 minutes more. Split into cups, and serve.

Nutrition:
Calories 310, fat 3g, fiber 5mg, carbs 12mg, protein 22mg

Traditional Beef Kebabs

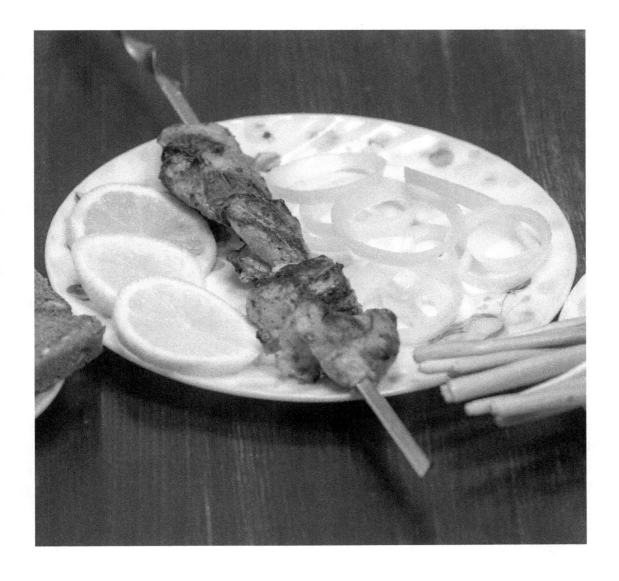

PREP TIME: 10 MINS

COOK TIME: 1 HOUR

SERVINGS: 4

Ingredients
- 12 ounces of white potatoes, cut into 1-inch pieces
- 2 teaspoons of grapeseed or canola oil plus 2 tablespoons, divided

- 1 small sized onion, finely chopped
- 1 pound of lean ground beef
- 1 large sized egg, beaten
- 1 medium sized red bell pepper, finely chopped
- 2 cloves garlic, minced
- ¼ cup of all-purpose flour
- 2 teaspoons of garam masala
- 2 teaspoons of ground pepper
- 1 ½ teaspoons of ground coriander
- 1 teaspoon of ground ginger
- ¾ teaspoon of kosher salt
- Fresh cilantro for garnishing

How To:
1. Add 1 inch of water to a medium saucepan inclusive of a steamer basket. Bring to a boil over a high flame. Add the potatoes and let the cook until tender (around 20 mins). Remove the potatoes, drain the water, then put the potatoes back in the pan. Cook until dry (around 2 mins). Transfer to a serving bowl and mash delicately with a potato masher. Then, let cool for about 10 minutes.
2. Meanwhile, warm 2 teaspoons of oil in a large non- stick skillet over medium flame. Add onion and cook, stirring often, untill soft (4-6 mins). Transfer to the bowl with the potatoes. Add red meat, egg, bell pepper, garlic, flour, garam masala, pepper, coriander, ginger and salt. Mix along with your arms until nicely combined.
3. Preheat oven to 400 tiers F. Line a baking sheet with foil.
4. To make every kebab, use your fingers to roll 1/4 cup red meat into a 4-inch-lengthy log. Make it more firm by pinching the ends to form a compact torpedo. Repeat to make 15 kebabs.
5. Wash and dry the skillet. Heat the final 2 tablespoons oil within the skillet over medium warmth. Cook half of the kebabs, without moving them, until lightly browned and crispy (1-3 mins). Transfer to the prepared pan. Repeat with the final kebabs. Bake until an instant-read thermometer registers 160 F (approx. 8-10 mins).
6. Garnishing with cilantro.

Nutrition:
Calories 310, fat 4g, fiber 6mg, carbs 12mg, protein 14g

Beef & Cabbage

PREP TIME: 30 MINS

COOK TIME: 1 HOUR

SERVINGS: 6

Ingredients
- 2 tablespoons of pickling spice
- 1 ¼ teaspoons of salt
- 1 teaspoon of dry mustard
- 3 pounds of boneless beef roast, cut it into 1 1/2-inch pieces
- 2 tablespoons of canola oil
- 2 cups chopped of yellow onions
- 1 ½ pounds of carrots, cut into 1 1/2-inch pieces
- 12 ounces of baby red potatoes
- 4 cups of low-sodium chicken broth
- 1 small head green cabbage, cut into 8 wedges
- 2 tbsp of chopped fresh dill
- 5 tablespoons of sour cream
- 3 tablespoons of prepared horseradish

How To:
1. Process pickling spice in a espresso grinder or spice grinder till finely dusted, approximately 10 seconds. Combine
2. the dusted pickling spice, salt and mustard in a small bowl; set aside.
3. Select Sauté setting on a programmable pressure multicooker. Select High temperature setting and permit to preheat for three mins. Meanwhile, sprinkle red meat frivolously with half of the pickling spice combination.
4. Add one-0.33 of the red meat and a couple of teaspoons oil to the cooker; cook, turning the red meat occasionally, until browned on all sides, about 6 mins total. Transfer the red meat to a bowl; repeat the process twice the usage of the last beef and oil.
5. Add onions, carrots, potatoes, broth and the ultimate pickling spice mixture to the cooker, scraping the bottom of the cooker insert to release any browned bits.

Return the red meat (and any collected juices inside the bowl) to the cooker; stir to combine. Top with cabbage wedges. Press Cancel.

6. Cover the cooker and lock its lid in place. Turn the steam release manage to Sealing position. Select Manual/Pressure Cook putting. Select High pressure for 30 min. (It will take upto 10 to 15 min for the cooker to come back up to pressure before cooking begins.)

7. When cooking is complete, permit the pressure release evidently for five mins. Carefully flip the steam release manage to Venting function and let the steam absolutely escape (the go with the flow valve will drop; this will take 2 to a few mins). Remove the lid from the cooker.

8. Transfer the red meat and vegetables to a platter; sprinkle with dill. Stir together bitter cream and horseradish in small bowl; serve the sauce alongside the beef and greens

Nutrition:

Calories 321, fat 6g, fiber 4mg, carbs 12mg, protein 18g

Beef Fajitas & Peppers

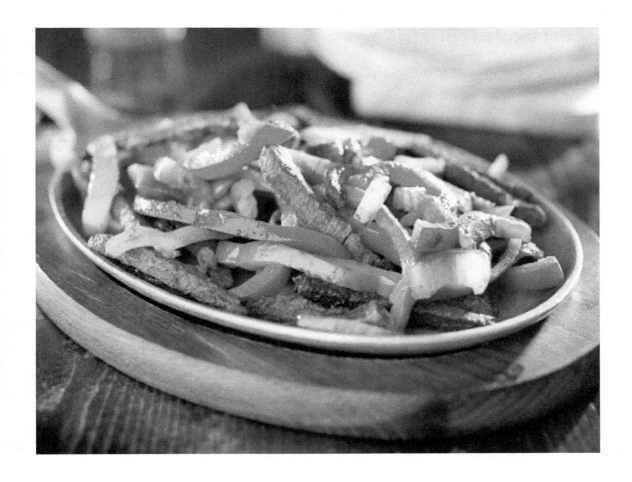

PREP TIME: 15 MINS

COOK TIME: 10 MINS

SERVINGS: 4

Ingredients

- Olive oil – 2 tsp. plus more for the spray
- Sirloin steak – 1 pound, cut into bitesize pieces
- Red bell pepper – 1, chopped
- Green bell pepper – 1, chopped
- Red onion – 1, chopped
- Garlic - 2 cloves, minced
- DASH friendly Mexican seasoning – 1 Tbsp. (or any seasoning without salt)

- Boston lettuce leaves – 12 for serving
- Lime wedges or corn tortillas for serving

How To:
1. Heat oil in a skillet.
2. Add half of the sirloin and cook until browned on both sides, about 2 minutes. Transfer to a plate.
3. Then repeat with the remaining sirloin.
4. Heat the 2 tsp. oil in the skillet.
5. Add onion, bell peppers, and garlic, cook and stir for 7 minutes or until tender.
6. Stir in the beef with any juices and the seasoning. Transfer to a plate.
7. Fill lettuce lead with beef mixture and drizzle lime juice on top.
8. Roll up and serve.

Nutrition:
- Calories: 231
- Fat: 12g
- Carb: 6g
- Protein: 24g
- Sodium 59mg

Slow Barbecue Brisket Sliders

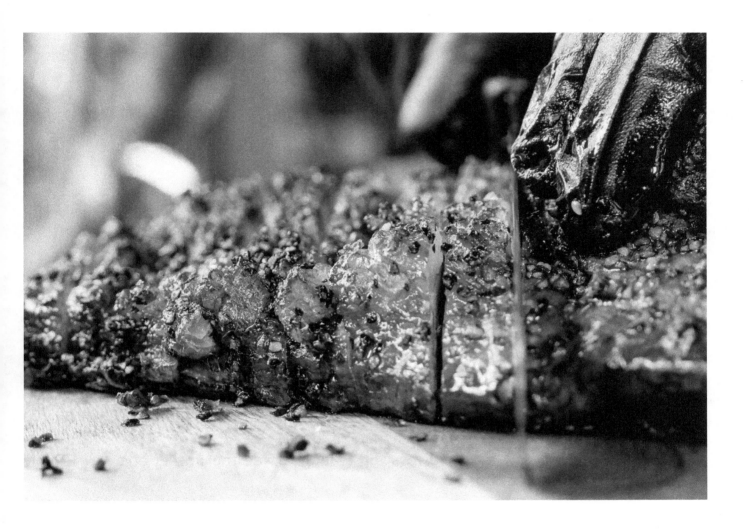

PREP TIME: 30 MINS

COOK TIME: 8 HOURS

SERVINGS: 6

Ingredients
- 2 chipotle chiles in adobo sauce, minced
- 1 ½ tablespoons of light brown sugar

- 3 garlic cloves, grated (about 1 tablespoon)
- 1 teaspoon of ground cumin
- 1 ½ tablespoons of olive oil
- 1 teaspoon of kosher salt
- ¾ teaspoon of black pepper
- 2 pounds of beef brisket, trimmed
- ¾ cup of water
- 2 cup of no-salt-added ketchup
- 2 tablespoons of lower-sodium Worcestershire sauce
- 3 tablespoons of apple cider vinegar
- 4 cups of shredded multicolored coleslaw mix
- 16 whole-wheat slider buns

How To:

1. Stir together the minced chipotle chiles, brown sugar, garlic, cumin, 1/2 tablespoon of the olive oil, 3/four teaspoon of the salt, and 1/2 teaspoon of the pepper in a small bowl. Rub all of this over the brisket.
2. Place the brisket in a 5- to 6-quart gradual cooker.
3. Whisk collectively the water, ketchup, Worcestershire, and a pair of tablespoons of the vinegar in a small bowl; pour over the brisket in the slow cooker. Cover and cook on LOW till the brisket is very tender, about eight hours.
4. Transfer the brisket to a slicing board, booking the sauce in the gradual cooker. Shred the brisket with 2 forks into bite-sized pieces. Return the shredded meat to the reserved sauce inside the slow cooker, stirring to combine. Just before serving, whisk together the ultimate 1 tablespoon every olive oil and vinegar and final ¼ teaspoon of salt and pepper in a medium bowl.
5. Add the coleslaw mix, and toss for coating. Divide the brisket and slaw evenly among the slider buns.

Nutrition:
Calories: 238, Fat: 7g, Carb: 14g, Protein: 27g, Sodium 167mg

Chapter 7: Fish & Seafood Recipes

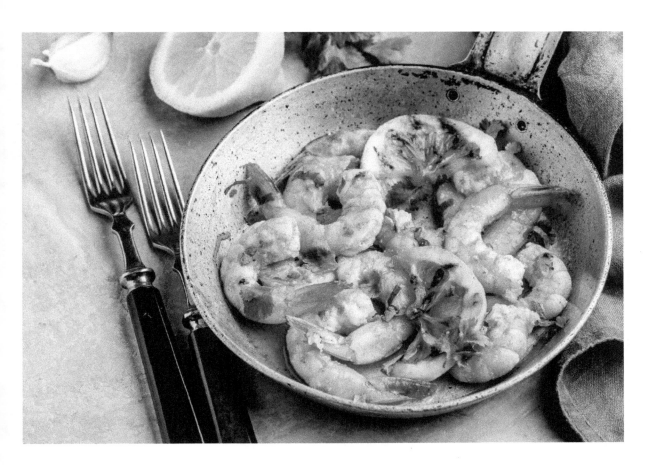

Spicy Baked Shrimp

PREP TIME: 10 MINS

COOK TIME: 8 MINS

SERVINGS: 4

Ingredients
- ½ ounce large shrimp, peeled and deveined
- Cooking spray as needed
- 1 teaspoon low sodium coconut aminos
- 1 teaspoon parsley
- ½ teaspoon olive oil
- ½ tablespoon honey
- 1 tablespoon lemon juice

How To:
1. Pre-heat your oven to 450 °F.
2. Take a baking dish and grease it well.
3. Mix in all the ingredients and toss.
4. Transfer to oven and bake for 8 minutes until shrimp turns pink.
5. Serve and enjoy!

Nutrition (Per Serving)
Calories: 321, Fat: 9g, Carbohydrates: 44g, Protein: 22g

Shrimp and Cilantro Meal

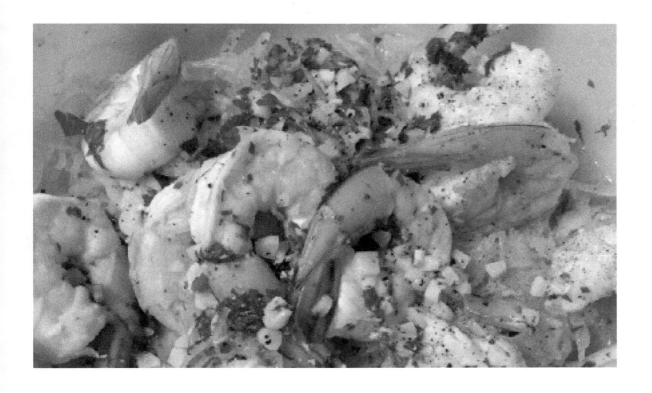

PREP TIME: 10 MINS

COOK TIME: 5 MINS

SERVINGS: 4

Ingredients

- 1 ¾ pounds shrimp, deveined and peeled
- 2 tablespoons fresh lime juice
- ¼ teaspoon cloves, minced
- ½ teaspoon ground cumin
- 1 tablespoon olive oil
- 1 ¼ cups fresh cilantro, chopped
- 1 teaspoon lime zest
- ½ teaspoon sunflower seeds
- ¼ teaspoon pepper

How To:

1. Take a large sized bowl and add shrimp, cumin, garlic, lime juice, ginger and toss well.
2. Take a large sized non-stick skillet and add oil, allow the oil to heat up over medium-high heat.
3. Add shrimp mixture and sauté for 4 minutes.
4. Remove the heat and add cilantro, lime zest, sunflower seeds, and pepper.
5. Mix well and serve hot!

Nutrition (Per Serving)

Calories: 177, Fat: 6g, Carbohydrates: 2g, Protein: 27g

The Original Dijon Fish

PREP TIME: 3 MINS

COOK TIME: 12 MINS

SERVINGS: 2

Ingredients
- 1 perch, flounder or sole fish florets
- 1 tablespoon Dijon mustard
- 1 ½ teaspoons lemon juice
- 1 teaspoon low sodium Worcestershire sauce, low sodium
- 2 tablespoons Italian seasoned bread crumbs
- 1 almond butter flavored cooking spray

How To:
1. Preheat your oven to 450 °F.
2. Take an 11 x 7-inch baking dish and arrange your
3. fillets carefully.
4. Take a small sized bowl and add lemon juice, Worcestershire sauce, mustard and mix it well.
5. Pour the mix over your fillet.
6. Sprinkle a good amount of breadcrumbs.
7. Bake for 12 minutes until fish flakes off easily.
8. Cut the fillet in half portions and enjoy!

Nutrition (Per Serving)
Calories: 125, Fat: 2g, Carbohydrates: 6g, Protein: 21g

Lemony Garlic Shrimp

PREP TIME: 5 MINS

COOK TIME: 5 MINS

SERVINGS: 4

Ingredients
- 1 ¼ pounds shrimp, boiled or steamed
- 3 tablespoons garlic, minced
- ¼ cup lemon juice
- 2 tablespoons olive oil
- ¼ cup parsley

How To:
1. If not yet boiled, boil shrimps (15 – 20 minutes)
2. Take a small skillet and place over medium heat, add garlic and oil and stir-cook for 1 minute.
3. Add parsley, lemon juice and season with sunflower seeds and pepper accordingly.
4. Add shrimp in a large bowl and transfer the mixture from the skillet over the shrimp.
5. Chill and serve.
6. Enjoy!

Nutrition (Per Serving)
Calories: 130, Fat: 3g, Carbohydrates:2g, Protein:22g

Chapter 8: Soup & Stew Recipes

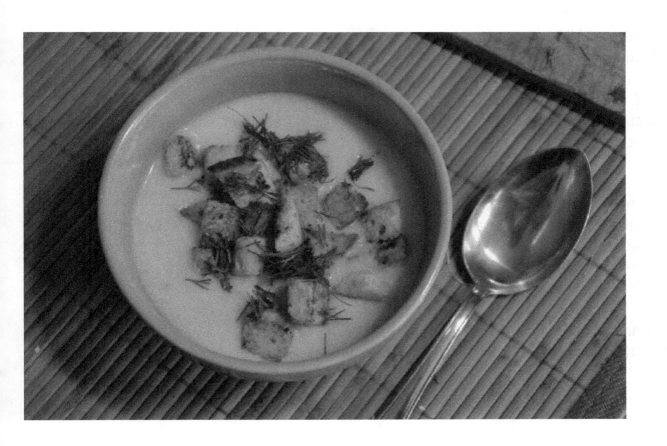

Chicken & Veggies Soup

PREP TIME: 5 MINS

COOK TIME: 30 MINS

SERVINGS: 4

Ingredients
- 2 tbsp. of olive oil 3 garlic cloves
- 1 onion
- 4 cups of low sodium chicken broth 1/2 cup of carrot, sliced
- 1/2 cup of parsnip, sliced
- 2 cups of a green collar, minced 1 can of black beans, drained 1/2 cup of seaweed (optional)

How To:
1. Simmer in the olive oil, garlic and onion blended.
2. Pour the broth and vegetables into the chicken, and turn to a boil. Switch to a simmer when boiling.
3. Keep on simmer until the vegetables are soft. Pour in the strained canned beans and optional seaweed when 5 minutes left to cook.

Nutrition:
Calories: 150, Fat: 6g, Carb: 24g, Protein: 9g, Sodium 160mg

Greek Lemon Soup

PREP TIME: 10 MINS

COOK TIME: 20 MINS

SERVINGS: 4

Ingredients

- Low-sodium chicken broth – 6 cups
- Long-grain rice – ¾ cup
- Chicken breast halves – 3, skinless, cooked and shredded
- Egg – 2
- Lemon juice – 1/3 cup
- Lemon slices, for garnish

How To:

1. In a saucepan, add rice and broth and bring to a boil.
2. Reduce heat.
3. Then cover, and simmer for 15 minutes.
4. Add chicken and simmer for 3 minutes more. Remove from heat.
5. In a bowl, whisk together eggs and lemon juice. Pour in 1 cup of hot soup broth, whisking continuously.
6. Add warm egg mixture to the soup pot and mix to combine.
7. Serve with a slice of lemon.

Nutrition (Per Serving)

Calories: 143, Fat: 16g, Carbohydrates: 6g, Protein: 3.4g

Mushroom Cream Soup

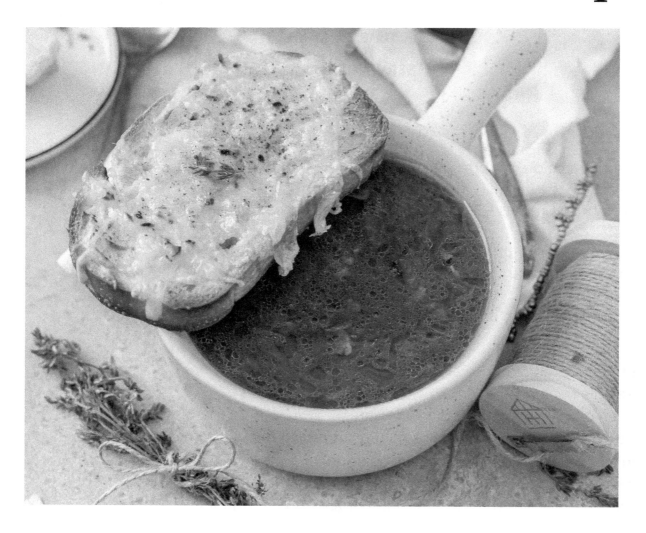

PREP TIME: 5 MINS

COOK TIME: 30 MINS

SERVINGS: 4

Ingredients

- 1 tablespoon olive oil
- ½ large onion, diced

- 20 ounces mushrooms, sliced
- 6 garlic cloves, minced
- 2 cups vegetable broth
- 1 cup coconut cream
- ¾ teaspoon sunflower seeds
- ¼ teaspoon black pepper
- 1 cup almond milk

How To:

1. Take a large sized pot and place it over medium heat.
2. Add onion and mushrooms to the olive oil and sauté for 10-15 minutes.
3. Make sure to keep stirring it from time to time until browned evenly.
4. Add garlic and sauté for 10 minutes more.
5. Add vegetable broth, coconut cream, almond milk, black pepper and sunflower seeds.
6. Bring it to a boil and lower the temperature to low.
7. Simmer for 15 minutes.
8. Use an immersion blender to puree the mixture.
9. Enjoy!

Nutrition (Per Serving)

Calories: 200, Fat: 17g, Carbohydrates: 5g, Protein: 4g

Lentil Soup

PREP TIME: 15 MINS

COOK TIME: 1 HOUR

SERVINGS: 4

Ingredients

- 1 onion, finely chopped
- 1/4 cup of olive oil
- 2 carrots, finely diced
- 2 stalks of celery, finely chopped
- 2 cloves of garlic, minced 1 teaspoon of dried oregano
- 1 bay of leaf
- 1 teaspoon of dried basil
- 1 (14.5 ounce) can of crushed tomatoes
- 2 cups of dry lentils
- 8 cups of water
- 1/2 cup of spinach, rinsed and thinly sliced
- 2 tablespoons of vinegar
- Salt to taste

How To:

1. In a soup pot, warm oil over medium heat. Add onions, carrots, and celery; cook dinner and stir till onion is tender.
2. Stir in garlic, bay leaf, oregano, and basil; cook dinner for two minutes.
3. Stir in lentils, and add water and tomatoes. Bring to a boil. Reduce heat and simmer for as a at least 1 hour.
4. When ready to serve stir in spinach, and prepare dinner table till it wilts. Stir in vinegar, and season to taste with salt and pepper, and more vinegar if desired.

Nutrition (Per Serving)

Calories: 371, Fat: 36g, Carbohydrates: 8g, Protein: 4g

Chapter 9: Salad Recipes

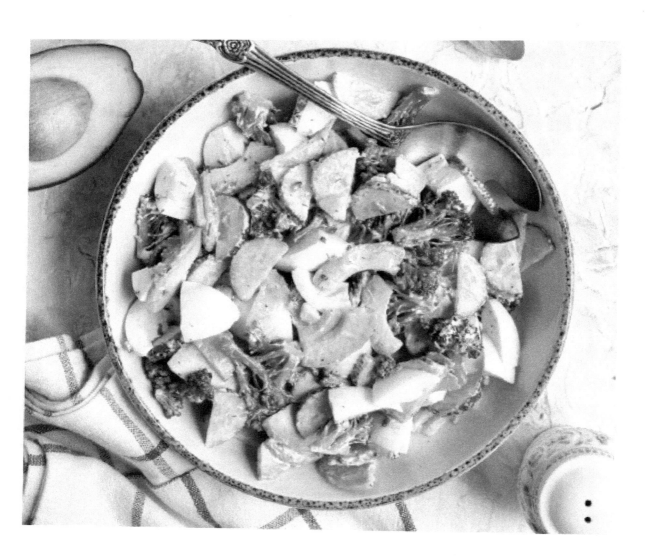

Spring Salad

PREP TIME: 10 MINS

COOK TIME: 0 MINS

SERVINGS: 4

Ingredients

- 2 ounces mixed green vegetables
- 3 tablespoons roasted pine nuts
- 2 tablespoons 5 minute 5 Keto Raspberry Vinaigrette
- 2 tablespoons shaved Parmesan
- 2 slices bacon
- Pepper as preferred

How To:

1. Take a cooking pan and when hot add bacon. Cook the bacon until crispy.
2. Take a bowl and add the salad ingredients and mix well, add crumbled bacon into the salad.
3. Mix well.
4. Dress it with your favorite dressing.
5. Enjoy!

Nutrition (Per Serving)

Calories: 209, Fat: 17g, Net Carbohydrates: 10g, Protein: 4g

Orange Salad with a taste of onion

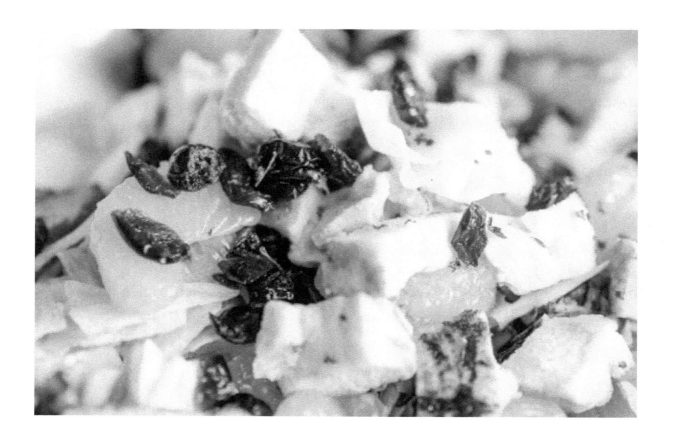

PREP TIME: 10 MINS

COOK TIME: 0 MINS

SERVINGS: 4

Ingredients

- 6 large oranges
- 3 tablespoons red wine vinegar
- 6 tablespoons olive oil
- 1 teaspoon dried oregano

- 1 red onion, thinly sliced
- 1 cup olive oil
- ¼ cup fresh chives, chopped
- Black pepper

How To:

1. Peel the oranges and cut them into 4-5 crosswise slices.
2. Transfer them to a serving bowl.
3. Drizzle vinegar, olive oil on top.
4. Sprinkle oregano.
5. Mix well.
6. Let it chill for 30 minutes. Then arrange sliced onion and black olives on top.
7. Sprinkle more chives and pepper.
8. Serve and enjoy!

Nutrition (Per Serving)

Calories: 120, Fat: 6g, Carbohydrates: 20g, Protein: 2g

Apple, Blue Cheese, and Pistachio Salad

PREP TIME: 10 MINS

COOK TIME: 0 MINS

SERVINGS: 4

Ingredients

- Apples – 3, peeled, cored and cubed
- Lemon juice – 1 Tbsp.
- Plain low-fat or 0% fat yogurt - 1 cup
- Cayenne pepper – ¼ tsp.
- Black pepper – ½ tsp.
- Blue cheese – 1/3 cup, crumbled
- Pistachios - 1/3 cup

How To:

1. Place apples in a bowl.
2. Then sprinkle with lemon juice.
3. Add yogurt and pepper to apples and mix to combine. Chill for 30 minutes.
4. Before serving, add blue cheese, and pistachios and mix.
5. Serve.

Nutrition (Per Serving)

Calories: 200, Fat: 8.5g, Carb: 25g, Protein: 8.5g, Sodium 200mg

Couscous & Vinaigrette

PREP TIME: 10 MINS

COOK TIME: 10 MINS

SERVINGS: 4

Ingredients

- Low sodium chicken broth – 1 ½ cups
- Olive oil – 2 Tbsp. divided
- Salt – ¼ tsp.
- Couscous – 1 ½ cups
- Orange juice – ¼ cup
- White wine vinegar – 2 Tbsp.
- Freshly ground black pepper
- Scallions – 3, finely chopped
- Fresh flat-leaf parsley – 2 Tbsp. chopped
- Sliced almonds – 1/3 cup

How To:

1. In a pot, add chicken broth, and 1 tbsp olive oil. Bring to a boil.
2. Add couscous, stir, and cover.
3. Remove from heat.
4. Let it sit for 5 minutes. Then fluff with fork.
5. Meanwhile, whisk together the remaining tbsp olive oil, orange juice, vinegar, ¼ tsp salt, and black pepper in a bowl.
6. Pour vinaigrette over couscous and mix well.
7. Add in herbs, scallions, and sliced almonds.
8. Season with more pepper and serve.

Nutrition (Per Serving)

Calories: 375, Fat: 15g, Carb: 52g, Protein: 9g, Sodium 230mg

Simple Side Salad

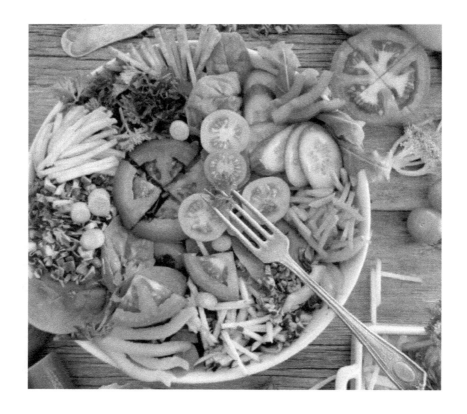

PREP TIME: 5 MINS

COOK TIME: 0 MINS

SERVINGS: 6

Ingredients

- 1 Romaine lettuce, chopped
- 3 Roma tomatoes, diced
- 1 English cucumber, diced
- 1 small red onion, diced
- ½ cup parsley, chopped
- 2 tablespoons virgin olive oil
- ½ large lemon, juice
- 1 teaspoon garlic powder

- Sunflower seeds and pepper to taste

How To:

1. Wash the vegetables thoroughly under cold water.
2. Prepare them by chopping, dicing or mincing as needed.
3. Take a large salad bowl and transfer the prepped veggies.
4. Add vegetable oil, olive oil, lemon juice, and spice.
5. Mix well to coat.
6. Serve chilled if preferred.
7. Enjoy!

Nutrition (Per Serving)

Calories: 200, Fat: 8g, Carbohydrates: 18g, Protein: 10g

Avocado and Cilantro Mix

PREP TIME: 10 MINS

COOK TIME: 0 MINS

SERVINGS: 2

Ingredients

- 2 avocados, peeled, pitted and diced
- 1 sweet onion, chopped
- 1 green bell pepper, chopped
- 1 large ripe tomato, chopped
- ¼ cup of fresh cilantro, chopped
- ½ lime, juiced
- Sunflower seeds and pepper as needed

How To:

1. Take a medium size bowl and
2. add onion, tomato, avocados, bell
3. pepper, lime and cilantro.
4. mix it all together.
5. Season to taste and serve chilled.
6. Enjoy!

Nutrition (Per Serving)

Calories: 126, Fat: 10g, Carbohydrates: 10g, Protein: 2g

Melon and Watercress become a Salad

PREP TIME: 10 MINS

COOK TIME: 0 MINS

SERVINGS: 2

Ingredients

- 3 tablespoons lime juice
- 1 teaspoon date paste
- 1 teaspoon fresh ginger root, minced
- ¼ cup vegetable oil
- 2 bunch watercress, chopped
- 2 ½ cups watermelon, cubed
- 2 ½ cups cantaloupe, cubed
- 1/3 cup almonds, toasted and sliced

How To:

1. Take a large sized bowl and add lime juice, ginger, date paste.
2. Whisk well and add oil.
3. Season with pepper and sunflower seeds.
4. Add watercress, watermelon.
5. Mix until all is well coated.
6. Transfer to a serving bowl and garnish with sliced almonds.
7. Enjoy!

Nutrition (Per Serving)

Calories: 274, Fat: 20g, Carbohydrates: 21g, Protein: 7g

Zucchini and Onions

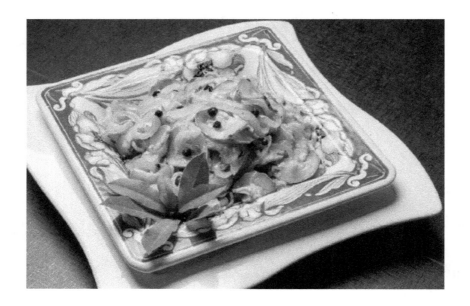

PREP TIME: 15 MINS

COOK TIME: 0 MINS

SERVINGS: 4

Ingredients

- 3 large zucchini, julienned
- 1 cup cherry tomatoes, halved
- ½ cup basil
- 2 red onions, thinly sliced
- ¼ teaspoon sunflower seeds
- 1 teaspoon cayenne pepper
- 2 tablespoons lemon juice

How To:

1. Create zucchini noodles (Zootles) by using a vegetable peeler and shaving the zucchini with peeler lengthwise until you get to the core and seeds.

2. Turn zucchini and repeat until you have long strips.
3. Discard seeds.
4. Lay strips in cutting board and slice lengthwise to your desired thickness.
5. Mix Zoodles in a bowl alongside onion, basil, tomatoes and toss.
6. Sprinkle sunflower seeds and cayenne pepper on
1. top.
7. Drizzle lemon juice.
8. Serve and enjoy!

Nutrition (Per Serving)

Calories: 156, Fat: 8g, Carbohydrates: 6g, Protein: 7g

Watermelon & Radish Salad

PREP TIME: 15 MINS

COOK TIME: 25 MINS

SERVINGS: 4

Ingredients

- 10 medium beets, peeled and cut into 1-inch chunks
- 1 teaspoon extra virgin olive oil
- 4 cups seedless watermelon, diced
- 1 tablespoon fresh thyme, chopped
- 1 lemon, juiced
- 2 cups kale, torn
- 3 cups radish, diced
- Sunflower seeds, to taste
- Pepper, to taste

How To:

1. Pre-heat your oven to 350 °F.

2. Take a small bowl and add beets, olive oil and mix to make sure everything is coated.

3. Roast beets for 25 minutes until tender.

4. Transfer to large bowl and cool them.

5. Add watermelon, kale, radishes, thyme, lemon juice, and toss.

6. Season sea sunflower seeds & pepper.

7. Serve and enjoy!

Nutrition (Per Serving)

Calories: 178, Fat: 2g, Carbohydrates: 39g, Protein: 6g

Chapter 10: Diner Recipes

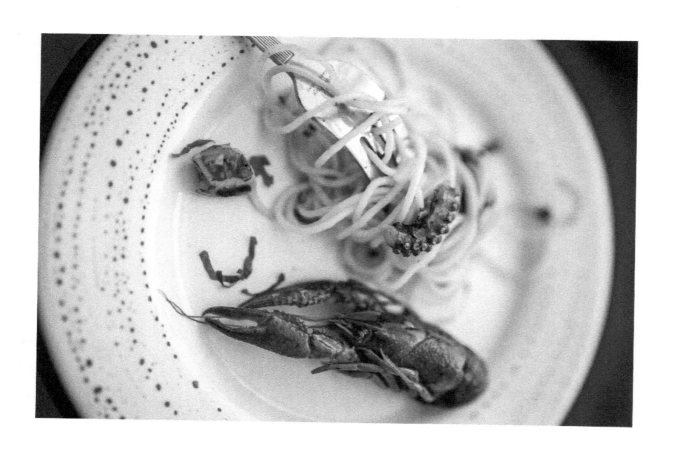

Almost Vegetarian Beef Meatballs

PREP TIME: 10 MINS

COOK TIME: 20 MINS

SERVINGS: 4

Ingredients

- ½ cup onion
- 4 garlic cloves
- 1 whole egg
- ¼ teaspoon oregano
- Pepper as needed
- 1 pound lean ground beef
- 10 ounces spinach

How To:

1. Preheat your oven to 375 °F.

2. Take a bowl and mix in the ingredients, and using your hands, roll into meatballs.

3. Transfer to a sheet tray and bake for 20 minutes.

4. Enjoy!

Nutrition (Per Serving)

Calorie: 200, Fat: 8g, Carbohydrates: 5g, Protein: 29g

Peppery wet Tenderloin

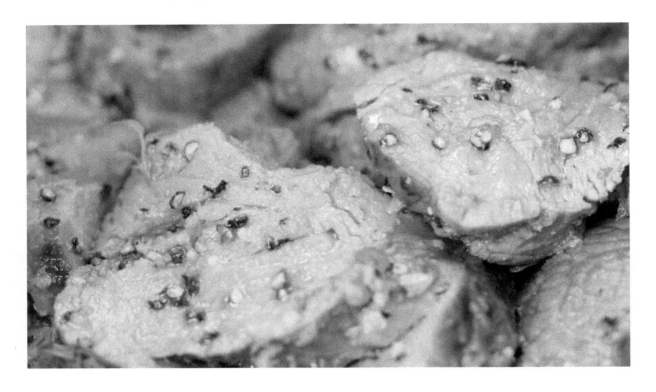

PREP TIME: 10 MINS

COOK TIME: 20 MINS

SERVINGS: 4

Ingredients

- 2 teaspoons sage, chopped
- Sunflower seeds and pepper
- 2 1/2 pounds beef tenderloin
- 2 teaspoons thyme, chopped
- 2 garlic cloves, sliced
- 2 teaspoons rosemary, chopped
- 4 teaspoons olive oil

How To:

1.   Preheat your oven to 425 °F.

2. Take a small knife and cut incisions in the tenderloin; insert one slice of garlic into the incision.
3. Rub meat with oil.
4. Take a bowl and add sunflower seeds, sage, thyme, rosemary, pepper and mix well.
5. Rub the spice mix over tenderloin.
6. Put rubbed tenderloin into the roasting pan and bake for 10 minutes.
7. Lower temperature to 350 °F and cook for 20 minutes more until an internal thermometer reads 145 °F.
8. Transfer tenderloin to a cutting board and let sit for 15 minutes; slice into 20 pieces and enjoy!

Nutrition (Per Serving)

Calorie: 183, Fat: 9g, Carbohydrates: 1g, Protein: 24g

Avo-Beef Patties

PREP TIME: 15 MINS

COOK TIME: 10 MINS

SERVINGS: 4

Ingredients

- 1 pound 85% lean ground beef
- 1 small avocado, pitted and peeled
- Fresh ground black pepper as needed

How To:

1. Pre-heat and prepare your oven to high.
2. Divide beef into two equal-sized patties.
3. Season the patties with pepper accordingly.
4. Broil the patties for 5 minutes per side.
5. Transfer the patties to a platter.
6. Slice avocado into strips and place them on top of the patties.
7. Serve and enjoy!

Nutrition (Per Serving)

Calories: 568, Fat: 43g, Net Carbohydrates: 9g, Protein: 38g

Surprising Beef Pot Roast

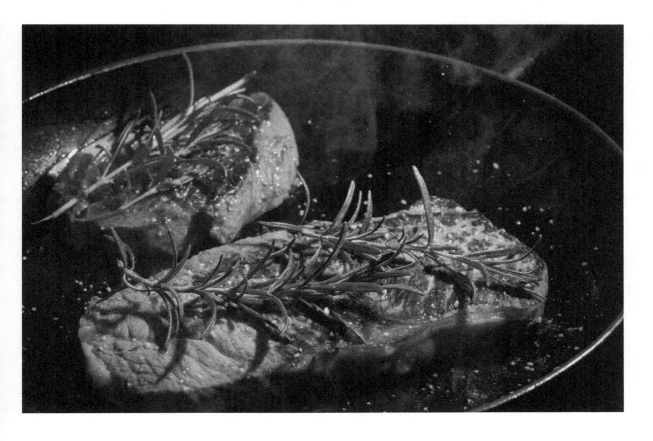

PREP TIME: 10 MINS

COOK TIME: 1 HOUR 15 MINS

SERVINGS: 4

Ingredients

- 3 ½ pounds beef roast
- 4 ounces mushrooms, sliced
- 12 ounces beef stock
- 1-ounce onion soup mix
- ½ cup Italian dressing, low sodium, and low fat

How To:

1. Take a bowl and add the stock, onion soup mix and Italian dressing.

2. Stir.
3. Put beef roast in pan.
4. Add mushrooms, stock mix to the pan and cover with foil.
5. Preheat your oven to 300 °F.
6. Bake for 1 hour and 15 minutes.
7. Let the roast cool.
8. Slice and serve.
9. Enjoy with the gravy on top!

Nutrition (Per Serving)

Calories: 700, Fat: 56g, Carbohydrates: 10g, Protein: 70g

Lying Mac and Cheese

PREP TIME: 15 MINS

COOK TIME: 45 MINS

SERVINGS: 4

Ingredients

- 5 cups cauliflower florets
- Sunflower seeds and pepper to taste
- 1 cup coconut almond milk
- ½ cup vegetable broth
- 2 tablespoons coconut flour, sifted
- 1 organic egg, beaten
- 1 cup cashew cheese

How To:

1. Preheat your oven to 350 °F.
2. Season florets with sunflower seeds and steam until firm.
3. Place florets in a greased ovenproof dish.
4. Heat coconut almond milk over medium heat in a skillet, make sure to season the oil with sunflower seeds and pepper.
5. Stir in broth and add coconut flour to the mix, stir.
6. Cook until the sauce begins to bubble.
7. Remove heat and add beaten egg.
8. Pour the thick sauce over the cauliflower and mix in cheese.
9. Bake for 30-45 minutes.
10. Serve and enjoy!

Nutrition (Per Serving)

Calories: 229, Fat: 14g, Carbohydrates: 9g

Epic Mango Chicken

PREP TIME: 25 MINS

COOK TIME: 10 MINS

SERVINGS: 4

Ingredients

- 2 medium mangoes, peeled and sliced
- 10-ounce coconut almond milk
- 4 teaspoons vegetable oil
- 4 teaspoons spicy curry paste
- 14-ounce chicken breast halves, skinless and boneless, cut in cubes
- 4 medium shallots
- 1 large English cucumber, sliced and seeded

How To:

1. Slice half of the mangoes and add the halves to a bowl.
2. Add mangoes and coconut almond milk to a blender and blend until you have a smooth puree.
3. Keep the mixture on the side.
4. Take a large-sized pot and place it over medium heat, add oil and allow the oil to heat up.
5. Add curry paste and cook for 1 minute until you have a nice fragrance, add shallots and chicken to the pot and cook for 5 minutes.
6. Pour mango puree in to the mix and allow it to heat up.
7. Serve the cooked chicken with mango puree and cucumbers.
8. Enjoy!

Nutrition (Per Serving)

Calories: 398, Fat: 20g, Carbohydrates: 32g, Protein: 26g

Spicy Chili Crackers

PREP TIME: 10 MINS

COOK TIME: 60 MINS

SERVINGS: 30

Ingredients

- ¾ cup almond flour
- ¼ cup coconut four
- ¼ cup coconut flour
- ½ teaspoon paprika
- ½ teaspoon cumin
- 1 ½ teaspoons chili pepper spice
- 1 teaspoon onion powder
- ½ teaspoon sunflower seeds
- 1 whole egg
- ¼ cup unsalted almond butter

How To:

1. Preheat your oven to 350 °F.
2. Line a baking sheet with parchment paper and keep it on the side.
3. Add ingredients to your food processor and pulse until you have a nice dough.
4. Divide dough into two equal parts.
5. Place one ball on a sheet of parchment paper and cover with another sheet; roll it out.
6. Cut into crackers and repeat with the other ball.
7. Transfer the prepped dough to a baking tray and bake for 8-10 minutes.
8. Remove from oven and serve.
9. Enjoy!

Nutrition (Per Serving)

Total Carbs: 2.8g, Fiber: 1g, Protein: 1.6g, Fat: 4.1g

German Eggplant Fries

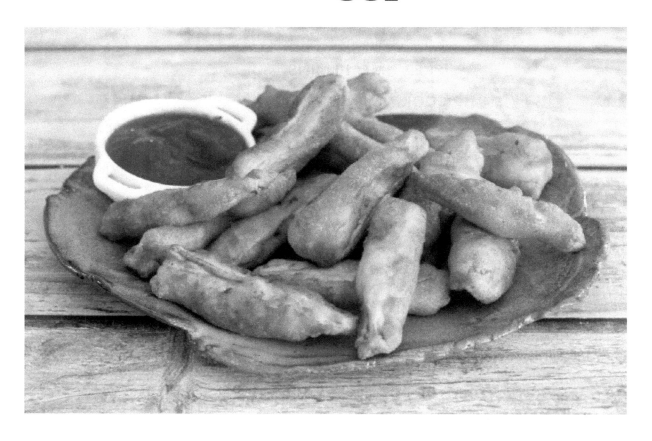

PREP TIME: 10 MINS

COOK TIME: 15 MINS

SERVINGS: 8

Ingredients

- 2 eggs
- 2 cups almond flour
- 2 tablespoons coconut oil, spray
- 2 eggplant, peeled and cut thinly
- Sunflower seeds and pepper

How To:

1.   Preheat your oven to 400 °F.

2.   Take a bowl and mix with sun-flower seeds and black pepper.
3.   Take another bowl and beat eggs until frothy.
4.   Dip the eggplant pieces into the eggs.
5.   Then coat them with the flour mixture.
6.   Add another layer of flour and egg.
7.   Then, take a baking sheet and grease with coconut oil on top.
8.   Bake for about 15 minutes.
9.   Serve and enjoy!

Nutrition (Per Serving)

Calories: 212, Fat: 15.8g, Carbohydrates: 12.1g, Protein: 8.6g

Cauliflower Steaks

PREP TIME: 10 MINS

COOK TIME: 25 MINS

SERVINGS: 4

Ingredients

- 1-pound cauliflower head
- 1 teaspoon ground turmeric
- ½ teaspoon cayenne pepper
- 2 tablespoons olive oil
- ½ teaspoon garlic powder

How To:

1. Slice the cauliflower head into the steaks and rub with ground turmeric, cayenne pepper, and garlic powder.
1. Then line the baking tray with baking paper and put the cauliflower steaks inside.
2. Sprinkle them with olive oil and bake at 375F for 25 minutes or until the vegetable steaks are tender.

Nutrition:

92 calories,2.4g protein, 6.8g carbohydrates, 7.2gfat, 3.1g fiber, 0mg cholesterol, 34mg sodium, 366mg potassium

Vegan Shepherd Pie

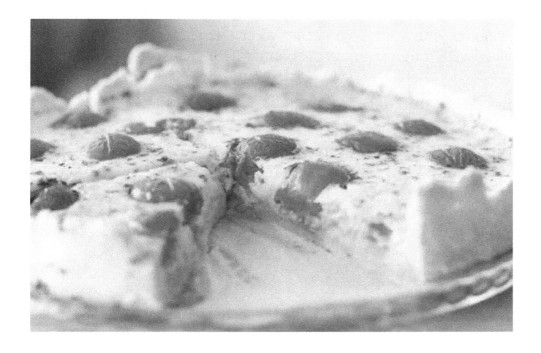

PREP TIME: 15 MINS

COOK TIME: 35 MINS

SERVINGS: 4

Ingredients

- ½ cup quinoa, cooked
- ½ cup tomato puree
- ½ cup carrot, diced
- 1 shallot, chopped
- 1 tablespoon coconut oil
- ½ cup potato, cooked, mashed
- 1 teaspoon chili powder
- ½ cup mushrooms, sliced

How To:

1.   In a saucepan, place the carrots, shallots, and mushrooms.

2. Add coconut oil and cook the vegetables until tender but not fluffy, for 10 minutes or until tender.
3. Then combine the cooked vegetables with the tomato puree and chili powder.
4. Move the mixture and flatten well into the casserole shape.
5. Comb the veggies with mashed potatoes after this. Cover the shepherd's pie with foil and bake for 25 minutes in the preheated 375F oven.

Nutrition:

136 calories, 4.2g protein, 20.1g carbohydrates, 4.9g fat, 2.9g fiber, 0mg cholesterol, 27mg sodium, 381mg potassium.

CPSIA information can be obtained
at www.ICGtesting.com
Printed in the USA
BVHW011527020321
601388BV00002B/114